—

www.30DayEvolveChallenge.com

Take time to write down your personal E.V.O.L.V.E. challenge.

"Your brain is the first muscle you must get in shape."

www.30DayEvolveChallenge.com

—

THE STRUGGLE IS REAL

Finally Break the Dieting Cycle,
Transform Your Mind and Body and
Evolve Into the Person You Have Always Wanted to Be.

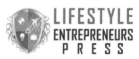

CHAPTERS

Testimonials

"The Struggle is Real" is exactly what people need when it comes to loosing weight. It's not about getting to the gym that's hard, nor is it about the lack of self-control. This book was extremely inspiring, motivating, and educating. I recommend anyone who has ever struggled, or is struggling with loosing weight, to read this book. It's guaranteed to make you want to do better for yourself."
~ *Bo Shin, Fitness Model, Bodybuilding.com and Labrada Nutrition Athlete*

Very inspiring and the fact that I'm able to relate is a plus. To hear how far both of you have come is testament that anyone can do it. You are both inspirations! Love and miss you and I'll be back at the gym soon. Signed up for the MS 150 bike ride next year!
~ *RuthPurcell*

I loved, change your brain to change your body. What Robby said in chapter 2, If you don't like the way you look or feel, then as long as you are breathing, you have an opportunity to change it. I love your, "struggle shield", and "what you eat in private, you wear in public". What really hit home for me the most was, Chapter 4, what you said, "The WHY lives deep within you, this is where you will find it, and once you own it, the decision to change it is the easy part. LOVE IT! And the back cover hit me like a ton of bricks!

~ Amy McCage Scales

For me "The Struggle is Real" will always be true. I've been over-weight for most of my adult life and just lived with that fact. But a health scare put me on a journey of living a healthier lifestyle by eating better and exercising. I was an emotional eater and always turned to food when feeling desperate. I never thought I'd enjoy exercising but I do now. I've been able to lose enough weight that both my health and self-esteem are back in check. Thanks to Karol and Bobby for sharing their stories. My struggle will always be there but knowing I won't be struggling alone makes the journey worthwhile.

~ Beth McDonnell

I'm half way through Chapter 3. And honestly. It hits the nail on the head with full force. It's absolutely true. Society wants results now and simply can not wait for them to happen. It's easier to make an excuse then progress. Like I always tell someone who says I want to do this or do that. While your in here making excuses someone else is out there making progress. Also the biggest problem I see when someone tries a diet is they want to jump in full force. You simply can not do that. You have to start out small. That's what I try to show the guys I work with. Cut out soft drinks. Drink more water and Gatorade. Walk 30 min a day. Then after a week add another 30 min. I see some cut everything and then run like 5 miles. The next 3 days they stop bc it's to much. But having someone to motivate you helps. But Karol you and Robbie definitely have something. And I'm so proud of you. I really am. I do look up to you as my motivation. Now more then ever.

~ Chris Breaux

As a female we almost all struggle with our weight unless you are genetically blessed and born thin. And in most cases, the struggle begins after child birth. I literally just had this conversation with my sister. I have 4 sisters. We were never taught to exercise. To this day only I and one sister exercise. Once I joined the gym in my 30's. I learned to eat healthy. I learned that it went hand in hand. I have since taught my daughter, No exercise no weight loss. We both love yoga.

~ *Becky Lachney Weeks*

These stories will encourage you to face your personal struggle, motivate you to create a plan, and inspire you to be successful. Karol and Robby are genuine and real as they share their stories and struggles and assure you that you are not alone.

~ *Cathy Guidroz*

1. I can relate a lot to your testimonies especially to Robbie as I always a chubby kid after 5th grade. I love the part about choices to be healthy or not. Especially the emotional eating and negativity section. The death of my father and a on going turmoil friends w/ benefits relationship has got me to that downward spiral but I will not let it break me down no longer, I am too good and came to far to gain the weight back. For me too my wake up call was biometrics and my wellness coach. Seeing those results in black and white made a ton of difference to get the weight off. Exercise is a great stress reliever for sure! My struggle is balancing it all together work, family, working out. :)

2. I love all the quotes and great examples to go along with it. Really enjoyed the knowledge area about weight watchers.

3. I wouldn't add or delete anything. A lot of information to get me focused on what I can do better in the struggle.

4. Loved the marathon story and I like both of your goal checklists. Robby's evolve is genius too.

Wish you both lots of success I think your passion and testimonies are so relatable.

~ *Kristina Kulp*

The Struggle is real is a great read; The success stories of these two amazing individuals, really helps the average person realize that we all indeed struggle. We all have had challenges and their stories help each of us to dig deep and realize that it's not always about the food & exercise but truly the emotions attached to our lifestyle, once we recognize it we can become successful in living a healthy life balanced and victorious. I will be sharing their book with my clients and am thankful for their dedication in Inspiring others.

~ *Yara Follette- Morgan*

The book connected with me on a very personal level. Often times the results of poor eating habits are discussed and addressed, but the underlying causes are not explored. Robby's personal journey helped me understand the root causes of my poor eating habits and how I can take a measured look each day and make healthy, educated decisions in my own life.

~ *Lanny Mixon*

The Struggle is Real is truly an amazing book. The authors really put their hearts into it. This book is packed with all the essentials needed for anyone looking to transform their life and take themselves to new levels. Very relatable, informative and highly recommended for anyone who is looking to get started or get back to where they once was at. You will be inspired knowing we all share the same daily struggles and together with this book we can overcome any of them

~ *Hughie Smith*

The book is inspiring to me on so many levels. Hearing the stories made me realize that I can achieve anything with a little will power and self motivation. It made me want to jump up and make a plan to change my lifestyle, right now! Waiting is out of the question!!

~ *Jillian Fisher*

The book is AWESOME!! I totally want every one of my clients to read that book. I have some clients that just can't commit and I think the book will help them so much. I also have clients who kick butt, totally beast mode, and bring the best condition they've ever been in to the stage for the first time in their life. But ... after the competiton is over and they can "cheat" a little, they keep cheating and it gets out of hand, and then they start getting depressed, then they give up and just keep binging and they never make it back to the stage. This post competition syndrome seems to mostly happen to the females but I have seen it happen to some guys. This book will help them keep sight of the true reason they started their journey in the first place.

~ *Denise Blackwell, Professional Physique and Bodybuilding Coach*

Here are my thoughts on the first three chapters of your book.. So far I love everything about the book and can't put it down. It's very inspiring and can't wait to read more because you have me wanting more. The most inspirational thing about the book is that of the reality and it's coming from a real place. It's not just about be ten pounds overweight, it's about two real people with the same real struggle millions of Americans have. I thought it was truly clever using each letter of the word struggle and connecting it to a word, each one of those words is truly inspiring, also the back cover poem (I think it a poem lol) have it as my screen saver love it!!! Y'all are doing/ did such a GREAT JOB!!!!!! Keep up the great work!

~ *Stephanie Soutullo*

So last night I finished chapter 2.... SPOT ON with all of the emotional, spiritual work that needs to be done.... TRUTH TRUTH TRUTH!!! I even said at my support group in August that I never really realized my emotional dependency on food until I couldn't binge.... I related to EVERYTHING about that!!!! Hoping to get a couple more chapters in this evening!!!!

~ *Tawny Freel*

We ALL have a struggle and you seek to empower, uplift and HELP! Thank you BOTH for being brutally honest and sharing your stories, AMAZING!!! If felt awash of emotions reading your stories, the RAW truth and vulnerability you share with your readers is courageous and encouraging.

~ *Yvette Forstall*

Dedication

This book is dedicated to the Old Us, to the ones who know
every day, the Struggle is Real.
This book is dedicated to everyone who struggles with their
weight and health.
This book is dedicated to the New YOU — Be Fearless, Be Fit.
How badly do YOU WANT IT?

Introduction

If you are holding this book in your hands, something inside of you is screaming for change. We all come from different backgrounds with different struggles, and every single one of us wants more out of this life. We all want to better ourselves and those around us, but our struggles build insurmountable barriers that prevent us from doing so. The struggles we face take on many different forms and come at us from every angle possible. We let those struggles keep us from becoming the person we have always dreamed we could be, and we make excuses to ourselves by saying, "If only I just wasn't dealing with _____ ." You can fill in that blank with anything that's holding you back, and many of us would need a lot more than just one space to fill in. At times it probably seems like you need an entire page to spell out all of the roadblocks.

For that reason we dedicate this book to you — everyone who knows all too well how "The Struggle Is Real" every day of your life. To those who have tried to lose weight but just couldn't stick to it and finish their goal. To all the yo-yo dieters of the world who want nothing more than to stop the vicious cycle of losing, then gaining, then losing again just to gain back even more than when you started. For those who struggle with emotional eating to ease the pain and fill the voids in their lives.

When we first sat down to write this book, we wanted to challenge the health and fitness industry by tackling an issue no one is really talking about. Every week there seems to be a new "Fad Diet" out that guarantees you will lose weight without ever leaving your couch or a new workout routine that proclaims all these incredible results without even changing your diet. The missing link that no one is talking about is also the biggest factor in determining your success or failure. What's inside your head and your heart truly determine the outcome of your life. We know from our own struggles that in order to change your body, you must first change your mind. The following chapters of this book will start you on the path to:

- Evaluate yourself
- Find and fix the problems inside your head and that are holding you back
- Peel back the proverbial onion to understand your emotional decision-making and make goal-oriented choices to set your heart's desires free
- Understand why it is important for you to make this change for you
- Develop an action plan and put it on paper. Set your goals, stick to them and achieve them to become the person you have always desired to be!

Our vision for writing this book is to tell our stories and share our beliefs and passion for a healthy lifestyle with as many people as possible. We have a deep desire to help people because we know the power of changing your life and seeing all the positive outcomes of your transformation. Everyone has the potential to do great things and accomplish their dreams if they want it badly enough.

We have written this book to open your mind and explore your heart to find what you really want to see change in your life. Every chapter develops the winning mindset by first getting rid of the negatives and then filling in the gaps with positive thoughts and affirma-tion through motivation. We challenge you to not only read the book but also participate in the challenges at the end of each chapter. Re-ally explore deep down inside of you and break down those barriers that are holding you back.

We are in this battle together against our struggles because united we are stronger. We can do this together because you shouldn't have to do this by yourself. Even if you feel all alone in your struggle, be-lieve us when we say you are not! After reading our stories in chapter 1, you will see just how much we both struggled for so long when change often seemed hopeless. But We were Stronger and we Did It. So can You.

Remember to tell yourself, "The Struggle Is Real, But I am Stronger!"

Chapter 1

Starting Point

Robby D'Angelo's Story

Hello, world, my name is Robby D'Angelo. I want to tell you a little about myself and my inspiration for pouring my life into this book. I believe we must understand the past in order to know what we want in the future. I can look back and know that I am admittedly 100% the product of my past and the choices I have made. As far back as I can remember I have always struggled with my weight and food. Some of my earliest memories involved being unhealthy and overweight. I can still vividly remember growing up with an insatiable appetite for all the foods that led me down that path.

My journey to become who I am today has more peaks and valleys than the Rocky Mountains. Growing up like most of America, I was never educated in making proper nutritional choices. Nor did it help that my mom's idea of a balanced meal was putting three different carbohydrates on a plate and calling it dinner. It wasn't her fault.

She was incredibly busy as she and my father were both high school teachers and coaches. She was just giving her boys what they wanted. By eating with my emotions, I developed a compulsive glutton eating disorder. Once I felt full, I would continue eating until it hurt. As a kid, I couldn't explain why I was this way with food. Many people say they are filling a void or food makes them happy. Being just a kid, I was unable to analyze why I binged to the point of misery. I now understand that I too was using food to compensate for something missing in my life.

In elementary school I was always known as the "fat kid" and often left out of the activities I could see everyone else enjoying. As a result I became very shy and introverted. I would often fake headaches and sicknesses to get my grandmother to come check me out of school early because I was so uncomfortable in my own skin around the other kids. I knew when grandma came to pick me up there would always be food involved. I knew exactly where she kept all the sweets that I could drown my emotions with. I was creating a pattern of emotional eating that I still carry with me to this day.

My entire family excelled in athletics. I grew up hearing stories, almost on a mythological scale, of how great an athlete my dad was in every sport imaginable. My mother, though, was arguably the better athlete, making it into her college's hall of fame as an outstanding basketball player. I also grew up watching my older brother follow in their footsteps by becoming a star athlete in every sport he attempted. I would watch him and say to myself, "One day I will be a great athlete just like him." Then there was me, the chubby kid who always lagged behind.

Most of the time I traveled with my family to my brother's golf tournaments and sporting events just to watch, and I could feel the envy building up inside of me. He had the talent and athleticism I desperately wanted. Growing up in that high-pressure environment, I became very insecure. I wanted more than anything to be the star athlete just like my older brother to make my parents as proud of me as I could see they were of him. I had a deep need for approval from my parents because of the insecurities I was harboring inside of me.

To this day, I still jokingly call myself the black sheep of the family. With everything I was dealing with, I had to find activities I could do by myself where I wasn't being compared to everyone around me. I began to be interested in art and would often spend hours sketching. It was my chance to mentally escape the real issues I was dealing with. It was something I could call my own that I could show my parents and say, "Hey, I'm talented too."

My insecurities weren't at all my parents' fault. I was blessed with some of the greatest parents anyone could ever ask for. Even though I was struggling on the inside and trying to hide it from them, they were always 100% behind me in every decision I ever made. They instilled in me values and qualities that I cherish and am so thankful for today. I know my drive and work ethic came from watching how hard they worked with all the long hours of coaching and how much they sacrificed to give everything they could to their three boys. I wouldn't be where I'm at today if it weren't for them pushing me to excel and dream big. Thank you, Mom and Dad, for what you sacrificed and poured into me as well as continuing to this day to my biggest fans! No words could express my gratitude.

The habits of my youth carried on until I was in seventh grade. Being fat and somewhat of an introvert assured that I never really fit in. I was struggling so much with my negative body image and insecurities that I was almost too embarrassed to be out in public, let alone try and make new friends. In order for me to find acceptance, I thought I had to become this overly nice guy. In my head I had to go above and beyond to please people because I had to make up for my negative body image. I would let people walk all over me and I would never even think of being assertive. I lacked confidence in who I was so I overcompensated.

I carried the "nice guy" mentality with me most of my life because, like most people, I wanted to fit in and be accepted. To me that was the only way I could. On one hand it kills me to think of the way I used to let people treat me because I didn't want to not fit in, but on the other hand, I am very appreciative that I went through this because it helps me stay humble and genuine when I tell my story. I know what you're going through and how badly you want to change but often feel like you can't.

Because of the values my parents instilled in me, I decided to change my life. It was because they believed in me and told me I could do anything I set my mind too. I was tired of being overweight and unhappy with myself. I was tired of not being able to be the real me because I was trapped within the walls of negativity I built all around me. I had developed so many coping and defense mechanisms to shield myself from the world around me instead of dealing with the problem at the root of it all—my weight. At this time of being sick and tired of being sick and tired, I finally made the decision to drop the weight.

In order for me to lose weight, I had to drastically change my eating habits and learn the discipline of making healthier choices. The transition from eating everything in sight to eating calorie-conscious foods was tough at first. I learned how to read food labels and understand exactly what I was putting in my body.

During my first weight loss, the only thing I knew about dieting was if I consumed fewer calories, I would lose weight. Breaking away from my gluttonous ways was tougher than I thought it would be. I often had this insatiable hunger that would just not go away even after a large meal. When the negative thoughts attacked me, they would bring on a plethora of negative emotions that left me feeling depressed and hopeless.

The mental battles one goes through are, in my opinion, the hardest part of any transformation. I battled those food demons on a daily basis. Even though I was only thirteen years old, losing weight was so important to me that I fought through the negatives and woke up every morning to eat a healthy breakfast and pack my lunch. Along with eating right, my love for sports was also coming into full swing about this time.

After I had lost a few pounds, I had the confidence I needed to really give sports the effort needed to excel where before I was just going through the motions because I thought it was what my parents wanted of me. During this weight loss I developed my love for football. It gave me another reason to eat healthier and get in shape. I knew if I wanted to be a star athlete like the rest of my family, it all started with my diet.

The greatest motivation for me was seeing the scale move. My parents were also great at providing support for my weight loss goals and helping me stay on track. My mom and I would sit down and plan my lunches before she went to the store so she could by me the healthier foods I needed. I was finally able to garner some of that attention I desperately sought after. I could literally see how proud my parents were of me when I made all district or received "Most Improved" awards.

One vivid memory I have is of my dad watching my game film and seeing me make a big play. I can still clearly see the prideful look on his face and hear how he bragged about me to the other coaches. In that moment I was finally proud of something I had done and finally felt accepted in my family. I wasn't just the black sheep anymore.

I got in shape for athletics and was finally healthy and fit. I was socially more acceptable and I was gaining happiness with myself. With the weight loss, I finally had the confidence in myself to break down those mental walls and start letting the real me out. I began to make friends, I actually fit in and for the first time I was truly happy with myself. I was finally able to be the person who had been trapped for so long he was almost lost. The positive self-image and confidence I gained during my initial weight loss was only temporary, though.

I came to a crossroads in my life. I was faced with one of the first major decisions I had to make regarding my future, and I struggled to find my answer. It had always been my dream to play college football like my dad and be a star athlete like my mother. I saw the way people revered them for their accomplishments and wanted to experience that. The problem was in the decision that lay in front of me.

I could continue my new healthy lifestyle, stay skinny and with tons of hard work, and have a small chance of playing on the next level. Or I could get big again and increase my odds of attaining my dream of being a college athlete. I put so much time and effort into losing weight, but I knew the probability of becoming a college athlete would be greater if I could drastically increase my size. I wanted both—to be lean and play football. The options in front of me were the two things I wanted the most at that point in my life, yet in my head the chances of having both were unlikely. I now know that I could have stayed healthy and still played college football, but I just didn't have the right knowledge base and took the easier path. In my head it would be a lot easier to just start eating again versus all the hard work it would take trying to keep my weight down.

I chose my dream. I went back to my ways of binge eating everything in front of me. I would eat anything I could get my hands on, just to gain weight for football. In my head I now had a purpose for my binge eating. It was what I had to do to chase my dreams. I took away the negative association with overeating and gave it justification. I still had zero knowledge into the proper ways to gain weight. I put on roughly twenty pounds each year of my high school career, and graduated at 6'2" and 285 pounds. Even though I was having huge success on the football field becoming a High School All-American my senior year, in my head I was once again dealing with overwhelming insecurities because of my weight.

As I started my college career, I was in a better situation but still eating unhealthy. I was built like a big, strong power-lifter but struggled to gain the weight I needed to in order to excel at my position. I played offensive line in college, mainly the center position, and if you look at the average weight of college offensive lineman played by giants of human beings, you would see most of the good ones weigh well over three hundred pounds.

Looking back it's crazy, but getting over three hundred pounds was a goal of mine. I thought it was what I needed to do to play. Even though I was a compulsive binge eater, I was constantly fluctuating about thirty pounds a year. I forced myself to be a compulsive glutton and would stuff myself full at every meal out of necessity. I would literally wake up every morning and make myself a 2,500-calorie protein shake, just to start my day. That's more calories than most people eat in an entire day.

I had the feeling of just leaving a buffet 24/7. I was constantly tired and lethargic and still expected to perform at a high level. Can you imagine how miserable it was trying to practice football everyday even though I had just put myself into a food coma? I thoroughly enjoyed my college football career and made some incredible lifelong friends, but there were certain aspects that I absolutely dreaded and the way I had to eat was one of them. Finding success on the field and being the massive strong guy on the team, I had many people watching at me and looking up to me. Experiencing that part was great, but inside all I could think about was wanting to once more get rid of the weight.

During my Junior year of football two major events happened that changed my outlook on life and I believe gave me the courage and strength to persevere through many of the challenges I would face in the future. Two weeks proceeding my first ever start as a college offensive lineman my little brother Anthony had major back surgery to correct a severe case of scoliosis and then Hurricane Katrina hit five days later. At the time I was living in Hattiesburg, which is sixty miles north of the coast, but do to a tornado that spun off from the high winds our house was damaged to the point of being unlivable. I actually had a tree laying diagnoly through my bedroom. I spent the entire rest of that football season living out of my truck and bouncing around from couch to couch of any teammate that would take me. I learned a lot through this experience. I learned how strong people can be when they are united toward a common goal and just how willing people are to help out those in need.

Five days before the hurricane hit my little brother underwent scoliosis surgery to straighten his back with titanium rods. He was 12 at the time and to see what he went through and the strength he displayed was extremely motivating to me. Everyday at practice I would write his initials on my taped wrists to remind me as bad as everything was, my little brother is displaying unshakeable courage through tremendous adversity. I wasn't able to be with him as much as I wanted to because I was in the middle of football season but I followed his progress with daily phone calls to my parents. I've never told him this but thank you for giving me strength through watching you overcome your surgery and the struggles that followed. I dedicated my junior season to him and it pushed me everyday to practice harder and give a little bit extra. I was hoping that my on-field success would in return help him get through the tough physical therapy of learning how to walk again.

As in high school, I again found success on the field, becoming an All-American at the college level and a finalist for the best player in the country at my position. The emotions associated with those achievements felt amazing, like I really accomplished something. During my senior season, there was something inside of me that kept resonating in the back of my head telling me I was just being who everyone else wanted me to be instead of being authentic to who I knew I was on the inside. I was one of the most recognized athletes on the team yet still felt empty inside.

My body had never gotten the proper nutrition it needed, and the years of all out abuse from practice and pushing myself in the weight room were now catching up with me. My body started physically declining and my knees started weakening. During my senior year of college football I was 6'2" and 305 pounds. I achieved my lifelong dream of playing college football but it came with a price. I endured four knee surgeries in a year along with numerous other injuries including a broken shoulder. My body was telling me "no more" and I came to the realization I had no chance of playing in the NFL. My dream was finally over.

As my senior year of football closed, I was dealing with never-ending pain, yet pushed myself to finish strong. Many mornings during the season, it would take me fifteen to twenty minutes just to get out of bed. If you wanted me to walk some stairs somewhere, first you'd better give me a little while to loosen my joints up. The week following my last game, I had double-knee surgery. At this point, for the second time in my life, I decided to get rid of the weight. Even then the only thing I knew about dieting was caloric restriction. At that time I was delaying the inevitability of the real world so I decided to stay in school for another year and a half to get my master's degree in business and finance. I also wanted to see what it was like to be a normal college student without all the responsibilities of football.

In order to attend grad school, I had to work my way through it, which did not leave me with a lot of time to work out like I wanted. I wasn't able to do a lot of cardio due to my knees. From just counting my calories, I lost almost one hundred pounds in one year... but I didn't look healthy. I had lost much of my hard-earned muscle mass from not working out like I used to. People would often come up to me and ask me if I was OK or possibly sick because they only knew me as this massive man. My whole life I had struggled with body image issues and now after losing the weight, I still couldn't lose the insecurities. I decided to really take control and understand how my body worked, which led me to really educate myself on all aspects of nutrition, lifting and the science behind getting healthy and fit.

I became extremely passionate about every aspect of living a healthier life. I became what I like to call a "health and fitness nerd." I had plenty of motivation to better myself because of all the negatives I built up inside of me through the years, but I didn't fully understand how to do it. I took my compulsive gluttonous ways and began to apply them toward something positive. I was tired of always filling the voids in my life with another negative decision that compounded into something even more detrimental to my health.

With this renewed spirit and motivation to succeed, I began to accumulate knowledge with the same insatiable appetite that I once applied toward food. A lot of times when we are searching for knowledge, we ask those around us. One lesson I learned from a mentor early on while in grad school was we cannot just listen to the loudest voice. We have to listen to the right voice. One person will say, "Stop eating carbs." Because they are skinny we just assume they must know what they are talking about, only to find out they were entirely wrong the whole time.

I was always a big believer in working smarter not harder. If I wanted to accomplish all my goals on this new journey of my life, I would have to reprogram my brain with the material it needed to make the best choices and stay motivated. I knew that in order to accomplish my future goals, I had to gain the knowledge of the proper way to do it. If I was going to apply myself to a goal, I wanted to go down the road with the best possible outcome. As I educated myself I became a part-time personal trainer just out of my growing love for fitness and so I could share my story to help others achieve their fitness goals.

The following years, from graduating college to where I am now, have been some of the toughest times of my life. I was not only continually struggling with my insecurities and a negative self-image, but now I was trying to find myself in the real world. As you have read, for most of my life when I set my mind to something I will do anything to accomplish that goal. However, at this point in my life, I was faced with learning the meaning of a new word that I did not have a lot of experience with— FAILURE.

I mentally struggled with failure for most of my twenties. I had just come down from the mountaintop of playing college football and now the struggles of the real world with real problems came full circle into my life. I thought I knew what career path I wanted but failed, which caused financial problems. I thought I knew who I wanted to spend the rest of my life with, but when that didn't work I looked at it as, "Once again I failed." "I'm just a failure" was a thought I couldn't shake.

On the surface everyone thought I was this exuberant, happy young man who really enjoyed life, but that was just a façade. I was actually in a dark place emotionally because of my failures and the fact I felt like I had lost my purpose in life. For the first time I didn't know what direction I was headed. Through all of this, I was also constantly battling with my emotional eating. I went back to binge eating to compensate for my emotions. I was in a vicious cycle—emotional eating then going back to eating healthy and working out until something else happened and it would start all over again.

My fiancé and I calling off our wedding was the final straw for me. After a few months of self-pity, dealing with the emotions of feeling like a failure and another knee surgery to top it all off, I decided to once and for all take control of my life. I had a good job and as always my family was my rock, so there were no excuses. The only thing stopping me from pursuing my passions in life was the negativity I built up inside of my own head. Enough was enough! The day I got off of crutches post knee surgery, my weight had ballooned back up to 240 pounds, the biggest I had been since my initial weight loss in college. I focused all of my energy into a renewed passion for all things health and fitness once again. Only this time I had learned from my roller coaster of a past and decided to not just diet again but make a lifelong commitment to health.

Two years later I have the best body I have ever had and accomplished things physically I never even thought were possible. I achieved a major milestone and something I never thought I could achieve—I have visible abs. I know it is just superficial, but to me it means so much more. It represents all the hard work and determination it took to take my 305-pound body down to 190 pounds. It represents the perseverance of making it through the struggle and the negativity inside of me.

Growing up we look at fitness magazines and aspire to have bodies like the people on the cover. As a crowning achievement, I did my first ever professional photo shoot for a supplement company that picked me to be one of their sponsored athletes. I can't lie to you and say I didn't have my insecurities standing in front of that camera, but seeing the pictures afterward made it all worth it. I actually just found out the ad for the supplement company will be placed in the number one men's health magazine in the market.

The meaningfulness behind this achievement is powerful to me. I used to look at these ads and say, "Man, I'll never have a body like that, but I sure wish I did." It's a great feeling of reward in yourself when you accomplish something you have always dreamed about. I finally am one of those "fit guys." I never thought that was possible. Also, to tackle another one of the demons (my negative body image) that I still struggle with, I am going to step out of my comfort zone and compete on stage in front of people and judges in a men's physique competition. I am doing this to challenge and overcome my negative body image. To go from someone who wouldn't take his shirt off on the beach to being judged by my body alone is a huge mental challenge for me. The competition is not for vanity so I can show off my body. I hope to mentally get past all the negativity surrounding the way I used to see myself.

Like anyone else I still struggle with controlling my emotional eating, and I do still have body image issues. But now I focus on turning the negatives into something positive. In the past, if I was having a bad day at work or was stressed over some issue, I would turn to food. Now I turn to the gym. Lifting weights in the gym has always been something I really enjoyed. No matter what was going on in my life, I could go lift some heavy weights and relieve the frustration. Presently, the gym is my therapy. For a little over an hour a day, I put my headphones on, crank them up and totally lose myself in the workout. Instead of giving in to my old ways when something negative happens and just harming my body, I have finally reprogrammed my brain to crave this positive action with actual lasting positive benefits.

Living a healthy life is a constant battle. Our lives get messy and it seems like everything is working against this new lifestyle. Usually our health is the first thing we put on the back burner so we can address the "more important" things in our lives such as work or family. If your health is really an important issue for you, like it was for me, you will make it a priority in your life. With small fluctuations here and there, I have managed to keep the weight off for eight years now and I am even more passionate about the health and fitness lifestyle than ever before.

Oftentimes when life becomes stressful I know that no matter what, I have an outlet where I can fully apply myself and release any negativity I have built up inside of me! Fitness has proven to be the one constant in my life, that when I make it a priority, everything else seems to fall into place.

I am often asked how I accomplished my transformation. So I tell my story with passion and conviction because I hope it inspires others. I have managed to lose and keep off 115 pounds. I say this in the most humble way possible because I know that if I can do it, so can you. For the first time in my life, I am 100% authentic to who I want to be and the feeling of joy that has come from that is unexplainable. I believe I am an eternal optimist and probably a little over enthusiastic at times, but for the first time I am honestly happy with where I've been and who I have become. I truly think every individual needs to feel good about who they are and where they are heading in life.

Before   **After**

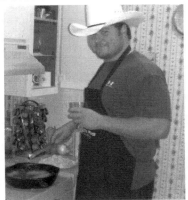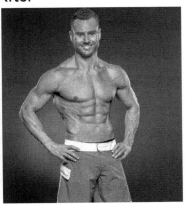

Karol Brandt-Gilmartin's Story

Growing up I was a very active child with fitness always at the forefront. I never thought of it as fitness because it was always so much fun. I have three older sisters—four girls, each almost a year apart in age—and the most amazing, loving, supportive parents. They are true role models for us all. My mother was a nurse and growing up was very focused on feeding us healthy foods from the pyramid of foods. She was very committed to making sure we ate very healthy, balanced meals. We had no soft drinks in the house and not a lot of processed sugars. Our desserts normally were fruit, Jell-O or pudding, and no chips or candy were in the house. She really did an amazing job of instilling balanced meals and nutrition within us all.

Both of my parents were extremely fit and active, with both of them playing tennis and racquetball at a competitive level too. They encouraged us to participate in all sports. We belonged to the YMCA and Green Acres Country Club growing up, which gave me a platform to be super active at a very young age. And, yes, we all went to dancing school. I think I liked it the most because I could watch myself dance and move in the mirror. I was into all sports imaginable—from CYO Cabbage Ball, swimming and diving to volleyball and track.

I loved being active and participating in as many sports as I could. But, my passions were gymnastics and dancing, and I excelled at them both. I rose quickly in the gymnastics ranks from classes to the gymnastics team, I was very strong and fearless, event back then, and wasn't afraid to try new gymnastic moves plus apply my dancing skills to gymnastics. One of my biggest inspirations, my coach Tara, used to take us into the weight room to lift weights. It was always so intimidating as there were always only guys in the weight room. My how that has changed! But, she would always do what she could to condition us physically to make us stronger and better gymnasts.

I had a bad break in my arm when I was in seventh grade and had to stop competing in gymnastics. But soon I realized I could do other things and still be able to participate in gymnastics and dancing. This built the platform for me to become a cheerleader for a very prominent high school with the reputation for the best cheerleading squad in the state. I so badly wanted to be on the squad. I tried out and I made it as one of the youngest cheerleaders to make the squad.

I was in heaven. Now I could do both and I focused all of my energy on being the best I could be. I had a male partner, as back then, it was female/male partners, especially for stunts. I loved being flipped around, twirled around and being part of this most amazing cheerleading squad. The only things I did not like were the weigh-ins. We had to stay within a certain weight range since we had boy partners and the guys were flipping us around, etc.

If you didn't make your weight, an alternate would take your spot. I think back to the stress this put on me to be at a certain number. I would eat salads and drink Tab two days out, so I could make my number and cheer. I was thick—all muscle. I was a gymnast so, my build was thick and strong, strong, strong. Too bad we didn't have BMI back then. I am sure I would have been given a few more pounds in consideration of my muscle, but that was not the case.

I could not and would not miss a game. That was all I wanted to do, so I dieted down even back then when I wasn't heavy. I even remember sitting in the attic with my cousin who wrestled and lent me a sweat suit so I could "sweat it out." I look at these pictures and say, "Boy, I was so skinny, so fit back then." But, the scale was becoming my enemy even at the age of fourteen. I found ways to ensure I hit my numbers every week, never to miss a game because of weight. It was one of my biggest struggles.

I also started coaching gymnastics, as I could not sit on the sidelines, knowing I could contribute to the development of the kids. I still wanted to hang out in the gym and be a part of the gymnastics team, somehow. This allowed me to still work out to an extent but also share my knowledge and experience with the younger kids and help develop them into their full potential.

Once I reached my college years, all the sports stopped. It was party time, and yes, I ate a lot more. I exercised a lot less but always seemed to manage keeping my weight in healthy check. I ran with my sister on the levy and still worked out at the YMCA. I did what I could to stay in shape, and I managed pretty well. I had put on a few pounds in my later twenties and when I got married, my husband and I walked almost every day to lose some weight. It worked, I was super thin and I felt great, but who knew it was the beginning of the yo-yo diet world for me.

A few years later, we divorced and I started a business with my then boyfriend. It was my dream to be in business for myself. And that was all I did for thirteen years—work, work, work and more work. No time for exercise, no time to cook, we ate out almost every day, twice a day, just to save time. I would try every now and then to lose weight. I'd lose a bit then gain it back. We travelled the countryside marketing our company and our events. We rode our motorcycle to some of the most beautiful, scenic places in the USA, and I would hate to take pictures because I would have to see myself in them. I would look at the pictures but just not me.

My self-image was at an all-time low. I felt so awkward, and my clothes were always too tight because I did not want to believe I was a size 22 pants and an XXL shirt. No way, not the cheerleader, not Karol. It was such a mental game and I was losing every time. It made me feel so ashamed, so ugly, and so insecure in every way. I had lost my sense of me, my self-worth.

My Disclaimer — I did not use any diet pill or have surgery to lose my weight.

In 2003, I joined Weight Watchers with a friend. The first year was good, but then we just let life get in the way. I just kept yo-yoing for several more years, losing thirty pounds, gaining fifty, losing fifty pounds, then gaining and settling with an extra eighty. I had lost all self-esteem and it was truly affecting all aspects of my life. I had no self-confidence and it made me feel so discouraged and most of all, hopeless.

Then in 2005, Hurricane Katrina hit and literally washed us away. We lost our business. We sustained major damage to our house and personally, the strain between us to decide what to save was the worst stress I ever experienced. We just could not endure it. We tried but the hurt was too deep. Everything we poured our hearts and sweat and money into, everything was gone and our city was in disarray. All I could do to numb the pain was to eat. I had stopped drinking and smoking on my thirtieth birthday, so I knew that was not an option. I did not want to take antidepressants and become addicted to living in a fog, so I ate, and ate, and ate and ate and ate. Food became my drug of choice and my addiction

I just ballooned up again, this time gaining even more weight, anything to numb the pain of losing everything. I had literally no foundation left at all and so much devastation all around. I moved around a lot. I lived in Galveston and then Clear Lake with my sister and then her friend. I was so embarrassed to come back home, so hurt and angry about what happened to us, and just felt lost and so alone, so hopeless. The only thing that eased my pain was food. I could find comfort in food, and boy, it just tasted so good.

I did, however, manage to dig deep and join a gym. I got a trainer by the name of Chris Cook and slowly but surely, with the help of him and my old weight watchers menus, I started to lose the weight and gain a bit of self-confidence. When I moved back to New Orleans in 2007, I had lost quite a bit of weight and was feeling better about myself. I got a job at Harrah's New Orleans and started reengaging with the work world. But inside I was still so distraught about what happened, I just kept eating to numb the pain.

I did not keep in perspective that when I came back, I put myself in a position to relive and open the Katrina wound again—the hurt, the loss, the devastation of losing my relationship, my business, everything. Once again, I turned to food. It was spring of 2008, and my life was getting ready to change again.

For many years, I would find excuses not to go out to social events because of my appearance and how it affected my self-esteem. Now you would meet me and say, "No way, not you!" But, YES, just like you, my self-esteem and my appearance made me want to crawl up and hide. However, my personality would not allow me to do that. I hated going out, watching people make comments about me to others or just look at me and say, "I did not recognize you." It would just rip my heart out and yes, drive me to eat (candy was my food drug of choice) even more.

Endurance—when I hear this word, marathon runners come to mind. They have to train to endure a physically grueling challenge. They have to go the distance and be mentally and physically prepared for the run, or they will not finish the race and cross that finish line.

When I got on the scale September 2008, I thought how did I let this happen to me again? How did this extra eighty pounds find me and how am I going to get rid of it for good? What a marathon to run, I thought.

Then, the reality of what I was doing to myself physically came about. I had an annual checkup with my wellness doctor at work. I dreaded going only because I knew she was going to say, "You are overweight and you need to lose weight." But this time it was so much worse than that.

We had taken blood the week before when we did my physical. We were reviewing the results, and I weighed in—eyes closed or backward on the scale, not to "see" the number—went into the room. The doctor came in with all of these pamphlets in her hand and I thought...hmmmm, these can't be for me, I am healthy. A "little" overweight but healthy. She stood next to me with her chart and literally shook my world. She said, "Karol, you are pre-diabetic. You have high blood pressure, and your cholesterol, the bad stuff, is super high." I looked at her in awe as thought she had the wrong chart. No way, not me.

She saw the shock on my face and asked, "Karol, why are you so surprised?" And I replied, "Because no one in my family has diabetes, high blood pressure or high cholesterol. My parents are super healthy and it is not hereditary. So, how is this possible? Are you sure you have my results?"

She looked me in the eye and grabbed me, moved me to the mirror, and said, "Karol, YOU have done this to YOU. You are severely overweight. You are 237 pounds and 5 feet 1 inch tall. All of these potential diseases you are looking at have been brought on by YOU. Look at yourself. This is the outcome of your choices."

I sat there in shock, sickened, saddened, embarrassed, humiliated, frustrated but most of all, it was the moment of acceptance. The doctor looked at me and said, "YOU need to fix YOU, so you will not have these health issues for life. As you said, these diseases do not run in your family. So, GO FIX YOU."

I left the clinic with the stark reality that yes, I had allowed my emotional eating and my lifestyle to control me and now I had put myself into a horrible health risk category. I left knowing the number on the scale, which sickened and saddened me. And, I left with the determination and willpower to say, "TODAY, I am going to take control of MY health, my life and I am going to CHANGE the course of my life to a healthy, fit lifestyle."

In 2008, some of my co-workers, my old WW friend, Sylvia, and I made a commitment to change our lives—for good. It was time for me to run my marathon of wellness. I went back to WW meetings in September 2008 —my Sunday morning class where the instructor, Pam Davis, and the attendees are very committed. They have been such motivation to me. They have kept my drive alive. The meetings helped me reframe my brain on how to deal with life's challenges without food and helped me change to a healthy, balanced lifestyle. The meetings enrich my mind, body and spirit. Every week I learn a new tool for success, and I have a huge toolbox now. When I left the first meeting, I was mentally ready to run that marathon.

And, with a new mindset, I did just that. I learned how to put myself first and take care of me. I began to prepare my meals every Sunday for the whole week. I joined a gym with my family and started to work out. I walked with co-workers in a few 5Ks and just kept believing and preparing, like the marathon runners do.

I joined an outside exercise boot camp in July. The first day I could not make it through the exercises. My face was as red as a tomato! But, I stayed the course and ten months into it, I felt like Superwoman… going faithfully three times a week at 6 a.m. I also hit the gym the other three days and tried and run once a week outside.

I found support with my parents as it truly takes a village sometimes to move the mountain—one step by one step at a time. My mom would help me cook, prepare and do meal prep each week for my lunch and dinner. My dad, my sisters and me would watch Biggest Loser every Tuesday night, and I would so relate. I would think this is ME, just not me on the TV show. Jillian and Bob's motivation, support and tough love to the people on the show inspired me in every way. I was building my toolbox of support and would go to it all the time for motivation, and it was working.

And, I found an amazing support at work. A colleague of mine, Jody Piper was struggling with her weight too. Remember, I live, eat and breathe in New Orleans, where, yes, we live to eat! She had moved from California and learned to enjoy New Orleans food as we all did. So, she too, made a commitment to get healthy and fit. So, we started bringing our lunch to work and every day for two plus years, we ate lunch, talked about recipes, exercise, and exchanged fitness and health tips every day. Jody, if I never told you, thanks for best mid-day therapy ever. It truly inspired me to see your commitment to changing your lifestyle and to live a healthy lifestyle. To this day,

Jody has kept her weight off and lives a very healthy, fit, happy life! We even had a few ladies who started doing Weight Watchers and we would cook recipes and bring the new meals to try. I felt good. I was coming back, my self-esteem was building, and by fall of 2009, I was actually feeling confident enough to yes to buy a new pair of "Skinny Jeans" and to be seen at concerts, festivals and social outings again. It felt GREAT to be out and for people to recognize Karol, me, for me and not have to be embarrassed over my appearance and have people judge me based on my size. I was beginning to feel fearless.

This was also when I started using Vision Boards. I would take all my fitness magazines, cut out and paste all the motivational quotes, photos of the fitness models, recipes, rock bands, hot dresses, skinny jeans all of the things I inspired to do and or be. This helped me visually see my transformation. I still use this today and encourage EVERYONE to have at least one vision board and keep it current. Put your pictures up there to remind you of your journey and appreciate how far you have gotten. I still have a pair of my size 22 women's pants as a reminder. I now fit into a 4 comfortably.

As a present to myself for my birthday in February, I signed up for the Rock and Roll Marathon in New Orleans. I knew I was ready to go the distance—13.1 miles. My goal was to run nine miles and walk the rest. I am so proud to say that I ran all 13.1 miles, and it was one of the most rewarding things I have ever done for myself. Running the marathon was a huge inspiration to me because that is how I refer to my journey of change—a marathon—and I stayed on course and finished strong! Jody was cheering me along the way with my parents and my sister. I am so very blessed to have had such an amazing support system to keep me believing that I can CONQUER this challenge. I can go the distance. The highlight of the race was afterward I met Maggie, one of the contestants from Biggest Loser. The connection we had and her inspiration just pushed me even harder. I too, wanted to inspire others to live a Healthy, fit lifestyle for YOU and put you first.

I submitted my story to Weight Watchers and in 2010 was selected as one of the Top 20 Role Models of the YEAR for Weight Watchers.

This was a BIG year for me, and another one of our WW attendees was selected too. It was such an honor for me to share my story and be selected nationwide as a Role Model. It confirmed that for me, I had to share my story on a bigger stage. I want to inspire everyone—to give hope that if you set your goals, you can crush them if you make good, healthy choices.

That was in February of 2010 and I never stopped running my heathy lifestyle journey. I worked with another trainer the next year, who helped me get leaner and stronger, the best I ever felt. By August of 2010, I was at my lowest body fat and leanest I had been in over twenty years. I felt great and it helped me build my self-confidence to a new high. I started seeing someone new in 2010 and he was into fitness big time—a bodybuilder who participated in shows. So, the pressure was on to stay fit. But, I was happy, so, I let my guard down just a bit. I ate ice cream with him, pizza with him, when he dieted down then ate up after, yep, I did the same thing.

He was a Chef, so he was always cooking something beyond delicious that might not be the healthiest for me. But, I worked out harder…did more cardio, trained more, whatever I could do to try and compensate for the food. But, I started to put some weight back on, and on top of that, my boyfriend used my weight gain against me and attacked me about my weight. Of course, that turned me back into my emotional eating again. It was my drug of choice, it was cheap, it tasted good and no one would "see" me do it.

I would eat in the car or late at night when he was asleep. It just once again filled the void and helped ease my pain. I look back now and think, it was only about ten pounds, but, boy did he punish me for my weight gain and I allowed it. I was emotionally being stripped of all that I worked to build up in myself. All of the hard work, exercise, meal planning, cooking, running a half marathon. Where did my willpower and self-esteem go? Where did my motivation to focus on ME go? Those ten pounds felt like one hundred pounds back on me. The weight of the world was on me and, this time, emotionally from someone else. I had allowed it. I had let my self-esteem, self-confidence and all of my good habits take second fiddle and I was now feeling it emotionally again. But, this time I knew what I had to do.

After a very volatile break up, I claimed my life back…again putting me at the forefront, letting nothing get in the way of my goal to fix ME forever. When I focused on me, the weight came off pretty quickly. I started taking spinning classes and enjoyed them so much, I got certified as a spinning instructor and taught spinning. I felt like I had reconnected with my coaching abilities and felt so invigorated in helping inspire others to change the course of their lives.

Once again I had reconfirmed my real calling, to spread the Word, the Struggle Is Real, but you can do it. I met a new guy at the gym (ironically), my Superman. He was brought in my life, I am convinced, to help me realize my self-worth and my self-confidence. He respected how hard I worked on me and would make me look at myself in the mirror and say, "Look at you, you look amazing. You have transformed your body and it shows. You work hard on you and it shows. Embrace it, enjoy it and use your talents to motivate others with your story." He will never realize the positive impact he made on my life by simply reinforcing my self-esteem and showing me I have the willpower to do anything. I can make decisions that will get me closer to my goals and change my brain to change my body. Very powerful words. Thank you, Superman, for all of your love and support and for making me look at myself in the mirror (even though I hated it, you made me learn to love it) and love me for me and to celebrate my successes.

I took a picture for Superman. I call it my FEARLESS picture, and I have enclosed it in the book. I still have it on my vision board today. I truly felt fearless in this moment.

As the New Year came, so did a new challenge. My sister was getting married in Key West in the summer and I had to be ready for six days in the sun and at a pool. So, I set a goal, six days, six bikinis, for all my struggles, to finally celebrate my successes and bask in the sun, literally.

I had started training with an amazing trainer, Maria, and was really focused on leaning out and building muscle and definition.

With the combination of spinning and training, anything was possible. Coupled with making great choices when it came to food, I was really seeing great results. It was almost effortless, easy for once, as I felt like all cylinders were clicking and I finally got it—eat healthy and exercise, every day, better choices will get me to my goal, and in my bikinis…yes, all 6 of them, one a day for Key West. I kept the course and when Key West Wedding week came, I never felt better. I truly felt fearless and confident wearing my bikinis. Feeling extremely fit and confident, my self-esteem was back for good and it was such a great feeling. I have several of those pictures on my vision board to keep me motivated every day to keep reaching for my goals.

Also, I had been introduced to this really cute, extremely fit guy, Colin, by a friend of ours named Mark. Mark was convinced that our passion for fitness, music and life were in parallel and we had to meet because we shared so many commonalities. That was in May of 2014 and when I met Colin, he gave me a hug and said, "You are so beautiful." I said thank you and for the first time it really did resonate. I was beautiful, me, inside and out, I finally felt good about myself and it was showing and attracting good, positive people in my life. Colin is a soccer coach, goes to Bikram Yoga (hot yoga, 104 Degrees in a room for ninety minutes) every day, and goes to the gym. I knew having someone who loves fitness as much as I do and who makes the time to take care of him that much and loves music as much as I do was a true fairytale story. Yes, once in a while, right in the middle of an ordinary life, love gives us a fairytale and that is what it has been since 2014.

Colin has me now going to Bikram Yoga with him. It is great to work out beside him, and I find my motivation in him and his commitment to a healthy lifestyle. I have surrounded myself with an amazing group of committed fearless ladies I work out with every week and an amazing trainer who gets me, sees my dedication and commitment, and pushes me harder at every work out. Zach has in this last year, transformed me to a leaner, fitter me than ever before. I have had some very powerful things happen in my life this year—some very sad and some very joyful. If I could have, I would have let my emotional eating join in on the fun, but not this time.

My job was eliminated after working with Harrah's for over eight years, and I lost my ex-boyfriend and business partner, Gary Sullivan, very suddenly just a few weeks before his daughter was to be married. I could have easily turned to food to numb the pain. But this time I realized I could handle these challenges without the candy bars, without the pizza, without the French fries. I knew I was strong enough and now had the tools I needed to work through my emotions and feelings without food. I actually worked out a bit more, played my music louder when doing my cardio and used the gym as a release for me, leaving me feeling much better about my choices and better equipped to handle the stressful situations. I will continue to do this moving forward and not use food as my crutch.

I also got married to Colin on July 19, 2015, at the Biggest Rock Wedding ever and I used this as another goal for me in my fitness journey. To feel fearless and 100% confident of me in every way. And, I did, we soooooo rocked the stage and had an amazing day. For the first time in over twenty years, I felt 100% confident. My self-esteem and self-confidence were soaring. I did it and I felt GREAT in my own skin, finally, and it showed. And guess what? I WANTED to see me in the pictures, finally!

The health benefits for me when I changed my lifestyle have been very noticeable to me. Physically, I get a full night sleep, my cholesterol is lower and my energy level is just through the roof! No health issues at all—no risk of diabetes, high cholesterol, nothing.

Mentally, I have retrained my thinking process when I eat and know that emotional eating is not the answer. The solution is eating healthy, exercising, learning to put yourself first, and telling yourself every day—GO THE DISTANCE, YOU CAN DO ANYTHING. It is not a selfish thing. It's the only way to succeed. You are worth the time you invest in yourself. Set a goal for YOU and make the right choices every day to get closer to your goal. Never lose sight of it.

I hope my story inspires and motivates you. Know that just like you, I struggle every day. But I know that the choices I make are mine and they will either get me closer to my goal or farther from my goal. I choose to reach my goal!

Your friend in Fitness

Karol Brandt Gilmartin

The most inspiring thing to me is knowing that I have positively inspired other people and they have joined the wellness journey and are now running the healthy lifestyle marathon with me. I have had several co-workers and friends join the gym, join Weight Watchers and eat healthier because of my total lifestyle change. There is no better feeling than knowing that my positive changes and results from Weight Watchers have directly affected someone's life for the better. I will strive to continue to inspire as many people as I can, sharing my marathon with them.

Before

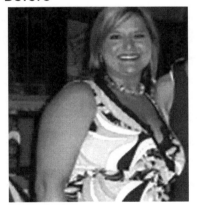

After

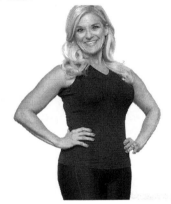

A Note from My Dad

Willpower. Willpower is made, not born. Sparked by desire and strengthened DAILY by repetition, anyone can develop willpower at ANY age.

I don't believe that willpower requires me to deprive myself of anything. I am simply making decisions to work with my mind and my body to achieve desirable goals. Developing that proper mindset is a gradual process. It does not happen overnight. Eventually, eating right and getting sufficient exercise become self-reinforcing and take on a life of their own.

The feeling that willpower necessitates certain unpleasant behavior and goes against one's nature is WRONG. Willpower is NOT a struggle against nature. It's working WITH nature to establish beneficial behavior patterns. Willpower is a set of learned habits and skills that can be applied successfully to every aspect of life. It is NEVER too late to develop willpower. How badly do you want it?

Dr. Lloyd Brandt Jr., Author

My dad wrote this and shared it with me more than ten years ago. Yes, I still have it on my vision board and read it regularly. He wrote this for him and for me, so I can remember that at any time, I can dig deep and find my willpower to accomplish anything I want. They are very powerful words and he still lives by them today.

Exercise 1: Write down your story. Try to gain an understanding of your past and what has led you to the point where you are today. You may have to write and rewrite it several times to fully explore all the facets that have made you who you are.

Chapter 2

Transformational Accountability

"Staring fear in the mirror was my turning point to saving my health."
~ Karol – at the turning point for change

Karol

The moment when Dr. Rose said, "Fix it," was a revelation for me. There I was, looking at myself in the mirror in disbelief. But seeing myself at that weight and hearing the results of my tests, I knew it was time to take responsibility for my actions.

At that moment, I owned it. I told myself that I was taking responsibility for all of my actions, all of the choices I made along the way to make me unhealthy and overweight. I realized then that through the stresses and emotional eating, I did this to me.

I embraced my struggle and finally held myself accountable held me, Karol accountable for where I was and in that moment. I took control of my actions, my life and I committed myself to changing the course of my life permanently. On that day, my life transformation began. I took control of ME and I owned it.

Dr. Rose made it sound so easy, just "Fix It." I left the office that day so very emotional but knowing food was not my option. My mind was made up and I kept telling myself, change, change, Fix It. I went home that night and told my parents the outcome of my test results. I shared my conversations with Dr. Rose. I told them I was holding myself accountable for my actions and I was ready to FIX IT! And, like many times before, both my mom and dad were 100% on board, committing to help me FIX ME in any way they could. Next, I went back to Weight Watchers with the commitment to hold myself accountable, chart all my food and activity, and learn as much as I could about my emotional eating. I wanted to APPLY this to my NEW healthy, fit, lifestyle. Next up, I joined a gym and a 6 a.m. boot camp. I had to have options for working out so I had no excuses for not working out.

This began my transformation for a better, healthier me and with all of the right tools, I knew this time I would FIX IT and fix it for good!

"Do not let your past dictate who you are, but let it be a lesson that strengthens the person you will become."
~ Unknown Author

We all have a story to tell. Every single person walking this Earth has experienced the roller coaster of life. We have all had times of great triumph or experienced unbelievable lows that we thought we would never recover from. Our pasts are what make us who we are. The past programs our brains and formulates many of the ways we think and make decisions. It also forms our self-image or how we feel about ourselves. You have to embrace your past and own it. The best lessons learned in life are often the ones we learn the hard way.

I know I tend to be slightly hardheaded and stubborn at times until I am forced to live through my bad decision.

Personal accountability is a lost way of thinking in our modern society. Many believe that in order to improve our country's low self-esteem problems we have to take personal accountability away from the bad choices we make. It has literally stripped you from any responsibility for your choices, leaving you with no consequences for your actions. Think about it. If you are depressed, there is a pill for that. If you are overweight, there is also a pill for that. It never seems to be anyone's responsibility. We are not saying that some do not have legitimate medical issues that require medicine, but most problems can be corrected by making the right choices and changing our thought processes. A recent study showed that those who read the American Medical Association's decision to call obesity a disease have a higher probability to choose high calorie foods and less likely to make healthy choices than those who did not read the article. Do not rationalize negativity in your life. Take accountability for it! Remember, this is YOUR LIFE and it is now time to take responsibility and be accountable for your actions.

Whenever we experience a problem or a setback, we have a hard time accepting the fact that a decision we made led to the current situation. The decision can be anything from the way we interpreted a situation or simply just not doing anything at all.

In order for you to change your life, you must first understand where you came from and what has brought you to your current situation.

"It is in the culmination of your choices that equals
the outcome of your life."
~ Robby

Robby

Embracing personal accountability is the first step toward changing your life. It is a harsh reality everyone has to come to grips with. You have to accept the fact that you are where you are because of you. Yes, we all have external factors and situations that affect us, but we are in control of how we react and deal with them.

One aspect of personal accountability is your reaction to outside influences. Taking control of you own choices is one thing, but being able to control your thoughts and emotions when external forces try and influence them is another. Every day whether you're at work, with friends or with family, not everyone is going to completely understand and support your goals and ambitions.

Your reactions to other people's decisions also play a part in your daily life and choices. Many people have told us time and time again, "There's no way you can do that." When I first started my transformation I just wanted to lose weight, but then after a significant amount of weight loss, I set a new goal of wanting visible abs. When I voiced my goals to people, I would often hear something along the lines, "You used to weigh over three hundred pounds. There's no way you can do that." Well I accepted that negativity as a challenge. My internal "I'll show you" mantra kicked in and it gave me the added motivation I needed to take my transformation to the next level.

Besides negative people, we are also surrounded by a multitude of stimuli on a daily basis—from the constant barrage of food commercials to walking into a convenience store and seeing those junk food aisles, the food TV networks, and everywhere on social media. Food porn is alive and well, and yes, we hate food porn!

Why? Because the Struggle is Real!

Life is never stagnant. It is constantly evolving and changing. Every day is different and presents its own set of challenges. Often we can let our surroundings and past control the way we act and feel about ourselves. You must have a paradigm shift that is positive and goal oriented. When your belief system is positive and strong enough, you will find that many of the problems you were having in the past due to outside influences simply do not affect you anymore. Instead of that way you used to think of it as a problem, now you have to see it as a challenge that you will overcome. Remember, you have no control over the outside world, but you are in 100% control of YOU.

You have to change the way you process information in your head.

When people process outside information and form reactions, they do so based on their belief system. Two people can see the same exact situation in two completely different ways. We all have some sort of negative baggage inside of us that influences our thoughts. We deal with negativity about our body image, our intellect and many other things. Changing your personal belief system is one of the first steps to changing your life. You have to believe you are worth the positive outcome of your new journey. You have to believe you can accomplish anything you set your mind to.

The key to handling negative baggage is to embrace and learn from your past. In my life the lessons that have had the biggest impact on me are the ones I have learned the hard way. The struggles in our lives are what makes us better, stronger people if we take them on with the right mindset. In school we often don't understand why we have to take so many history classes. The real purpose is so we can learn and grow from the past. We learn that things like dictatorships, greed, and so on have all led to negative consequences, so in the future we know not to embrace those ideals. We also have to put that concept to work in our personal lives.

Personal growth is not just reading and learning new material that will make you a better person. It's also learning from your past and growing as an individual. Many individuals are content with where their lives are and simply do not choose to better themselves. If you are reading this book, chances are you are not like them. You grow from the implementation of attained knowledge. We must learn how to be better people and make better decisions, but we also must take action steps. The best diet in the world will not make you lose weight unless you actually follow it.

How does your decision affect you emotionally?

You emotional well-being plays a pivotal role in the decision-making process. When you are trying to accomplish a goal but make a decision that sets you back, it is depressing. You work so hard to make the right choices, when you have a moment of weakness it emotionally hurts. When you are in a happy positive mood, you are more inclined to make the right choices that align with your goals.

When you're emotional healthy, you are in control of YOUR emotions and behavior. It has to all work together. Your emotions drive your actions and your actions drive your emotions. So, when you are healthy emotionally, your behavior shows it. These choices and your actions will lead you closer to your goal. You have to address your emotional struggles just as much as your food struggles.

Self-image is a large determining factor in the choices you make. The beliefs that are engrained in your subconscious lead you toward decisions without you even realizing it. In order to move forward, you must first remove the negative weight that burdens your thought processes. Your past does not equal your future. Self-fulfilling prophecy states that you become what you believe. If you believe you're genetically overweight, you will just use that as an excuse for why you cannot lose weight. When most people want to make a change in their life, they rely solely on willpower. But as we all know, willpower is a limited commodity. You have to first change your belief system and your self-image. You must believe and think into fruition what you want to accomplish. It takes practice and, like any other body part that you want to improve, it takes work.

When starting the journey to this new you, the very first step is self-evaluation. In order to make a decision that is best for you, you must change your beliefs and your attitudes. In order to help someone make the best decision for themselves, you need to explore their attitudes and beliefs toward factors of that decision. If you are starting a journey to a healthier, stronger version of yourself, it has to become aligned with your emotions and desires. If you do not truly desire to be healthier, you won't be. If you are not in an emotional state to fix your physical self, start by problem solving what's inside of you because that is where it all starts. You have to dig deep inside of you and root out the negativity and the insecurities. A physical change simply cannot come unless you mentally change along with it. In order for you to change, it must come from the inside.

Every one of us has incredible potential once we make the decision and follow it up with conviction. Many emotional and metal factors can hold someone back from making this positive change. Many lack internal control, suffer from low self-esteem, or say, "This is just the way I am. I can't change." The good news is—it's all reversible. While it may take some time and effort, you can completely change your self-image into the person you have always dreamed of becoming. Positive self-image works just like any muscle in your body—the more you work it, the stronger it will get. It's vital you start with a positive self-image knowing today is the start to a better, stronger, healthier (inside and out) version of yourself.

For both of us, we know personally that we are at our weakest when we are feeling down. We tend to make bad choices that can compound into other bad choices if we're not careful. We call this the negative spiral. As we mentioned earlier, unhealthy options are always around us and they are toying with our emotions. Emotionally, we start thinking about how good that cheeseburger will taste or how satisfying that bowl of ice cream will be, and that wreaks havoc on our emotional well-being. When you make a decision with negative consequences, it most often brings you down further, creating that negative spiral.

As society progresses we are becoming even more addicted to immediate gratification. We have forgotten what hard work and discipline are because we want it now. When your internal reward system is based off immediate gratification, you are going to have a hard time trying to change your life. With technology and the incredible speed at which our world works, we have everything at the click of a mouse or even as easily as picking up our phones. While this is very beneficial—and trust me, I take full advantage of it—it trains our brains to want things now. When we cannot get what we want out of a situation, we simply move on to the next because it did not immediately gratify us.

The human mind is one of the hardest things to change. You cannot simply decide one day to be a more positive person and expect that to last you the rest of your life. You have to constantly work on it even when negative situations present themselves. People who want to transform their mind and body want it to happen now.

"How come I haven't lost any weight? I ate a salad today for lunch."

"I worked out yesterday how come my biceps aren't growing?"

Remember it has taken your entire lifetime to form the present version of yourself, and you simply cannot change that in a day. Changing a behavior pattern or a thought process is far more difficult than formulating one for the first time. As humans we do not start each day with a clean slate of negative thoughts and feelings.

"Nothing in life worth having comes easy."
~ Unknown Author

Life is not easy. If your life is easy and you think you are doing just fine, then you are doing something wrong. Challenge yourself daily to become a better version of you. It will not come with immediate gratification, but it will also not come with regret. You will never hear anyone say they regret becoming a better person.

Many individuals who start a transformation of the mind and body are emotionally fine because they still have that fresh motivation pulsing through their veins. As time goes by and the initial motivation wears off, emotions want to take over. Your mind is constantly battling with your emotions. You know inside of you when you make a decision based on emotions versus one you took time to logically think out.

Our emotions play on our need for immediate gratification while our logic will make a decision based on long-term effects. When you are faced with a decision you know you shouldn't make, it is obviously not aligned with your long-term goals and you must step back and evaluate the emotions you are dealing with. Do I want to binge eat because I am stressed or depressed? Binge eating was always our drug of choice to cope with emotions. We still struggle with fighting back emotionally led bad decisions. That's why you hear everyone say #TheStruggleIsReal.

Emotions and desires often drive people's attitudes toward certain things.

We have to change the way people process information. When people process outside information and reactions, they do so based on their belief system. Two people can see the same exact situation in two completely different ways. We all have some sort of negative baggage inside of us that influences our thoughts. We deal with negativity about our body image, our intellect and many other things. Changing your personal belief system is one of the first steps to changing your life. You have to believe you are worth the positive outcome of your new journey. You have to believe you can accomplish anything you set your mind to.

Robby

We have all had body image issues at some point in our lives. For me, body image is still a constant struggle.

Growing up as the "fat kid" I never was comfortable in my own skin. I was always tugging on my shirt so it didn't show any fat rolls. I did not participate in some activities because I refused to take my shirt off. Males and females both struggle with body image issues. These are insecure emotions surrounding what we see in the mirror. Even those with the physiques you admire have their own insecurities regarding their bodies. Either they are not skinny enough, they do not have as much muscle mass as they want, etc. Just like us, they struggle too.

I shouldn't laugh but I find it a little comical when I hear someone say, "I have to get in shape before I can go to the gym." Isn't the whole purpose of the gym to get in shape? Some would say the current gym I work out in is hardcore or only for the advanced because a lot of power lifters and competitors work out in there. But inside you find a completely different environment. They offer beginners classes and their slogan is even:

"Everyone Starts Somewhere"
~ Richard Hawthorne, Southern Elite Gym

The challenge is overcoming those body issues. If you don't like the way you look and feel, as long as you are breathing you have an opportunity to change. Negativity associated with body image can lead to some just giving up. The good news is—it's all reversible. While it may take some time and effort, you can completely change your self-image into the person you have always dreamed of being. Positive self-image works just like any muscle in your body, the more you work it, the stronger it will get. It's vital you start with a positive self-image knowing today is the start to a better, stronger, healthier (inside and out) version of yourself.

Personal growth is not just reading and learning new material that will make you a better person. It's also learning from your past and growing as an individual. Many individuals are content with where their lives are and simply do not choose to better themselves. If you are reading this book, chances are you are not like them. You grow from the implementation of attained knowledge. We must learn how to be a better person and make better decisions, but we also must take action steps. The best diet in the world will not make you lose weight unless you actually follow it.

The biggest thing you can do is stay in a positive mood and stay focused on how good it will feel to accomplish your goals. When you are feeling down, it is time to do some self-exploration to understand what put you in this mood. This will help you determine what you can do to prevent it from happening in the future. Understanding your triggers—whether ones that bring you down or ones that build you up—will help you stay in the right emotional state to facilitate accomplishing your goals.

When starting the journey to this new you, the very first step is self-evaluation. In order to make a decision that is best for you, you must change your beliefs and your attitudes. In order to help someone make the best decision for themselves, you need to explore their attitudes and beliefs toward factors of that decision. If you are starting a journey to a healthier, stronger version of yourself, it has to become aligned with your emotions and desires. If you do not truly desire to be healthier, you won't. If you are not in an emotional state to fix your physical self, start by problem solving what's inside of you because that is where it all starts. You have to dig deep inside of you and root out the negativity and the insecurities.

A physical change simply cannot come unless you mentally change along with it. In order for you to change, it must come from the inside. Every one of us has incredible potential once we make the decision and follow it up with conviction. Many emotional and mental factors can hold someone back from making this positive change. Many lack internal control, suffer from low self-esteem or say, "This is just the way I am. I can't change."

It's time to take responsibility of YOUR actions, just like Karol did when she walked out of the doctor's office that day and took responsibly of her poor eating habits and lack of exercise. The only person who can change you is YOU!

> *"My past has not defined me, destroyed me, deterred me, or defeated me;*
> *it has only strengthened me."*
> *~ Dr. Steve Maraboli*

The powerful thing about the past is it is just that—your past. Every day you wake up with a clean slate and the opportunity to put your past behind you and become the person you have always wanted to be.

Exercise 2:
Now take time and think back to some of the life-changing decisions you have made. What led you to that decision? What emotions were you dealing with? Write them down

and really explore what in your life has most controlled your decision-making process.

Chapter 3

Real Power of Choices

Robby

I needed to understand the power of my choices to make a change.

When I started my journey to become a healthier me, I did not fully understand how to do it. I just knew I had a deep desire to become the best version of myself I could. I began immersing myself into the world of health and fitness and I learned the power of every individual choice I made. Even the smallest of decisions helped me move forward or put me two steps back. At first making the healthier choices was hard because of my previous lifestyle and being busy while I worked my way through graduate school.

Growing up in a very competitive athletic family, I was instilled with certain qualities at a young age that really have paid off for me. The one quality that has helped the most is defining a goal and then doing what needs to be done to achieve that goal. I knew if I wanted to excel as a college offensive lineman, I was not only going to have to perform on the field but do the small things right even when no one was looking. I applied this deeply engrained mindset to the new goal of losing all the weight I had gained playing football to become a healthier, fitter me. Once the choice was made, I had to align my day-to-day choices with my new goal.

I started small by making better food choices and avoiding the foods I knew I would get in trouble around. We are all human and have urges to make the wrong decisions, but if you keep your goal in mind and are conscious of how these choices will affect you, it becomes easier to stay strong. As you will learn, the more you make the right choices, the easier they become. You get to the point where you thrive off doing what's right.

Decisions, Decisions, Decisions… Every morning upon waking, you are faced with thousands of choices from brushing your teeth to deciding what to eat for breakfast. The decisions you make, no matter how big or small, affect every outcome and direction of your life. Most decisions we make in life happen at the subconscious level, meaning you do things without even thinking about them. The power of your choices has made you who you are and will also determine who you become. Right now you could be doing a million different things, but you are making a choice to read this book. Just as in chapter two, you have taken responsibility for your past choices. You must now own every choice you make from here on. You are in control. You have the power to drastically alter your life and it all starts with a decision.

Three words that changed my life:

"Everyone makes choices."
~ *Coach Sykes*

No other statement in my life has had the impact those three words had. They explain everything. They take away all problems and excuses. If you do not like your current situation, make the choice to change it. Coach Sykes was one of my football coaches in high school and it drove me nuts every time he would say this because it's so true.

I grew up playing football in Southern Mississippi where oftentimes the heat index was well over one hundred degrees and the humidity was topped out at 100% as well. It literally felt like you were trying to practice football in a piping hot bowl of chicken noodle soup. What Coach Sykes did was take away all the negativity and excuses with those three simple words… "Everyone makes choices."

"But, Coach, it's too hot to practice today," or, "My legs are too tired to keep running," and the endless other excuses anyone who has ever coached knows all too well. Coach Sykes' answer was always the same. "Everyone makes choices." And sometimes he would even elaborate if he was in a good mood. He would follow up with, "You can go inside right now. You could be at home in the A/C watching TV and eating bonbons, but you made the choice to be out here and practice." The next time someone is complaining to you or making excuses, simply utter those three magical words and watch the expression on their face.

I tell this story because we often do not own our decisions. We are quick to blame outside circumstances and other variables when ultimately everything is our own decision. You have to be conscious of the decisions you are making. If you keep making decisions the way you always have, how do you expect anything to change?

We all know that the best way to make a decision is to focus on the long-term effects and not on what is pleasurable now. Many choices we are faced with on a daily basis are made based on what we want now. The taste of the cheeseburger versus the effects on your health. Go lay out in the sun without sunscreen to get a tan versus the damage it is doing to your skin. Focusing on what is immediately pleasurable often leads to negative outcomes, and the problem with this method of making choices is it can have a snowball effect. The bad decision you just made was really satisfying, so the next time you are presented with that problem, you are more likely to think about the pleasure you derived from it versus the long-term effects.

The choices we make daily have permanent consequences whether we want to think about them that way or not. One of my favorite quotes that reminds me of this is:

"Every choice is either a step closer or a step farther from your goals."

We have to retrain our brains to focus on the long-term effects of each individual decision. A long-term focus further allows us to align our choices with our goals. If your goal is to get off blood pressure medication, the decision to go the buffet is counterproductive. Everything inside of you may be saying, "Go eat it… One time won't hurt you…" As we often say, the brain is a muscle just like any other in the body, and with work it gets stronger. The more you can focus on what you want for your future self instead of what you want right now, the easier the choices become with time. The more long-term decisions you make, the easier the next one is, and so on. Healthy people do healthy things because they enjoy being healthy. It's a mentality they form. A choice that is more enjoyable is easier to make. You have to enjoy the choices to become healthier.

The way you look is a by-product of the way you feel. Where most people fail in a health transformation is their initial motivation and mindset. They start simply to fix a problem area or the way they look. The problem is they often don't do it for long because it's just superficial. It does not have a deeper meaning. When your back is against the wall and you are forced to make a choice, that decision is more likely to become permanent.

Those who change for lasting health benefits often stick to that decision a majority of the time. We have learned that those faced with health challenges often make decisions to improve their health and the majority actually follow through. Why? Because they are forced to make the decision not just for vanity but also for their health. It is not just a temporary plan they start to lose a couple pounds and look better. They make the decision to be healthier because it will hopefully prolong their lives.

The decision to become healthier starts within. Physical change only happens when change happens mentally. Becoming physically attractive is merely a by-product of this journey and not nearly as attractive as the confidence that comes with the transformation. When you start this journey to health, people will begin to see the changes from the inside out. They will notice that extra bounce in your step and the new smile on your face.

Conquering your mind and body is one of the most fulfilling things any individual can do. The reason why is because it is not an easy thing to do. It's going to be hard and at times, The Struggle Is Real. But because you are making this decision internally first, those struggles are not going to seem so insurmountable.

People often make decisions for different reasons even when given the same circumstance and possible outcomes. So to truly nail down how and why people make decisions, we have to dig deeper into their internal passions and motivations. The one definitive reason that leads to most decisions is outcome based. People weigh various outcomes and make a decision based on them. So when it comes to your health, you are more likely to stick to a decision with a long-term positive outcome of you becoming a healthier more confident version of yourself.

Preconceived notions and biases also play a large role in the decision-making process, especially when those two are both negative. The individual is not likely to pick the best outcome based on that thought process. We all have thoughts and emotions associated with the way we feel about ourselves. Self-image is a large determining factor in how we make decisions. If you personally see yourself as a motivated individual who enjoys taking on new challenges, you are more likely to follow through on the goals you set for yourself. On the other hand, if you view yourself as someone who just is bad at everything and never lucky, or you're just not good enough, that is going to be the way you approach your goals.

Many individuals let their self-image make decisions for them without even giving it a second thought. In the past you have made so many decisions based on the negativity surrounding your self-image that it has just become normal to you. In the south we call this "Stinkin Thinkin." We all know those people who go through their entire life without even the idea of a positive thought. Saturday Night

Live used to run a very funny skit called Debbie Downer. No matter the situation or what positive activity was going on in her friends' lives, she always found the negative in it. She always pointed out what could go wrong or what negative circumstance could arise from the topic at hand. Stinkin Thinkin is precisely the self-image and mindset we have to rid ourselves of before we can do anything to improve our current situation.

Decisions are often made after someone explores all possible outcomes and weighs all the available information they have. The problem with health decisions is either someone doesn't have the education to make an informed decision, or if they go and try finding information, they are bombarded by information—often that conflicts with one another—and it all becomes very confusing and overwhelming.

Uncertainty with the outcome of a decision is part of any decision-making process. When we stand at the fork in the road, we have to make a choice. When you are uncertain where each road leads, making the choice of one over another becomes more difficult. The good news is uncertainty is all but removed from the question to become healthier or not. We have plenty of evidence to the benefits of living a healthy life versus continuing our unhealthy ways. The uncertainty in this equation comes in the how you are going to make this journey but not why you should start. We will talk later about the "how," but now we are going to focus on the initial decision.

The decision-making process is very complicated with many different variables to consider, but with focus and willpower they become simple. A simple decision coupled with high motivation has been shown to increase the likelihood of making the best decision that will last. When making a decision to start your health transformation, it is a very simple choice—to be healthy or not. People often overcomplicate the decision when trying to understand the thousands of diets and workout plans out there. They become overwhelmed with all the variables and possible outcomes.

What if this happens?

What happens when I do this?

Am I strong enough to do this?

Do I deserve this?

Am I worth the sacrifices I may have to make?

What will my family and friends think?

Will they support me?

They get overwhelmed and almost into a state of shock to the point they never get started. Questioning a change is normal, and if we don't think about all the factors that go into a change, we may not make the right decision. A decision to be a healthier you is not complicated at all. You want to, you need to and you will. Make the decision to be healthier and do it! One large often-insurmountable challenge to a lot of people is they seriously fear change. The negatives associated with all the "what ifs" absolutely terrify them. People often fear having to give up something in their lives they really enjoy or giving up something that provides them with a sense of security. The thought of the dieting and exercising process can be really intimidating because of all the unknowns.

Science has proven that when you make a decision without thinking of all the surrounding variables and "what ifs," it is easier to make the decision that is best for the long term. A simple choice is the easiest to make. If you can take away all the negative thoughts inside your head surrounding your choice to be healthier, you are far more likely to follow through with the decision.

Yes, there will be setbacks and lessons learned along the way, but the key is to move confidently in the direction of your goals with an unwavering belief system. If you keep two things in mind during your transformation, there is no stopping you. You must constantly remind yourself of why you wanted to change in the first place and how good it's going to feel to reach your goals. When you lose sight of those two things, you lose sight of your key motivating factors. Times are going to be tough, the struggle is real, you are going to have times of weaknesses (I know I sure do). But if you keep your key motivating factors in the forefront of your thought process, there really is no stopping you. You can accomplish everything you want and then some!

A health and fitness transformation involves every aspect of your life, so the decision-making process must become more conscious rather than subconscious. You have to actively engage yourself in every decision you make. This is often very difficult to do because of the pace most of us live our lives. We are in a non-stop rush every single day with work, family and obligations. Every day, we have so many decisions when it comes to food choices. It has become sensory overload, from the baked goods in the glass counter when we get coffee to the food we were raised on. And for us, that meant being raised on the best in world-famous food, Southern Food, from New Orleans and the Gulf Coast.

Be mindful of EVERYDAY choices by really taking the time to think your decisions through.

"Great things are done by a series of small things brought together."
~ Vincent Van Gogh

Making the right choices that are aligned with your goals will build strength through willpower. That strength and willpower will help future choices become easier to make. As others see you making the right choices, they will begin to understand how serious you are about reaching your goals. Making the right choices can be hard at times especially when dealing with negative thoughts and emotions. That is why when making choices you must keep your goals in mind.

Make conscious choices every day. Keep in mind that the choices you make now shape your future. Understanding that, you now can fully control the outcome of your life. We all have negatives in our past, but the key is to live in the present with your eyes on the future. The past you does not define the future you. The choices you make today can and will change your life for better or for worse.

Everything that goes into your body and every calorie you burn is a choice you make. If I eat this cheeseburger, it's going to take me an hour on the treadmill to negate my wrong choice.

Once you understand where you are, you now can align your life's compass with your goals. Every choice you make now has to align with your goals. For most people it takes twenty-one days to form a new habit. Making healthy choices—whether it be working out or eating—becomes easier the more you make them. Willpower is a muscle and the more you work it the stronger it becomes. In our lives we are faced with many struggles that will try to pull us away from our goals, and our willpower keeps us on course.

The major problem with willpower is it is a limited resource. Only so many times can we use willpower to make the right decisions before we break. People are more likely to make the right choices when they have a full tank of willpower versus having to constantly use it with every decision made throughout the day. In order to preserve your willpower to times when you really need it, you should make many of your daily choices much easier.

Some simple ways to do this include:

- Remove tempting foods and drinks from your sight and out of your house if possible
- Pack your lunch and snacks for work
- Pack your gym clothes in your car so you can go straight from work or during your lunch break
- Pick a gym that is on your way home or more convenient for you
- Do not make your workouts longer or more complicated than they need to be
- Make sure your exercise routine is fun and enjoyable

Willpower's number one role is to control and overrule our emotions. Too many decisions that we make are based on emotions rather than a logical goal-in-mind thought process. Every time you make the right decision, to skip the cinnamon roll, to go to the gym, to get an extra workout in, that decision, that step, will affect your outcome. It will get you closer to your goal, and when making the right decisions every day, you will achieve your goal. Why? Because that's how WE did it, small steps, right choices, good decisions = ACHIEVING YOUR GOALS. And there is no better feeling that standing on top of the mountain, knowing that you are there because you made the right decisions.

When you make the bad choices, when you slip, when you cheat, when you celebrate with food, you're only bringing yourself farther away from your goals. When we are in the moment, we often do not think about the consequence of negative choices. It is important to understand consequences when you make both good and bad choices.

It seems that when we make the bad decisions, it sometimes happens because of our surroundings—whether the kids want ice cream on a hot summer night or your husband has a sweet tooth and can eat dessert every night in front of you—this is where the Struggle is REAL. But, YOU need to be selfish, put your Struggle Shield on and make the choice not to eat dessert with him every night. Make this choice for you to bring you closer to your goal.

> *"Winning is a habit. Watch your thoughts, they become your beliefs. Watch your beliefs, they become your words. Watch your words, they become your actions. Watch your actions, they become your habits. Watch your habits, they become your character."*
> ~ *Vince Lombardi*

We are all human and give in to bad choices every now and then, but the key is to understand what choices you made and how to fix them in the future. You have to make the right choices when nobody is looking. You are making this decision for you and no one else. The deeper the inner desire to change for the better, the easier it is to make the right choices. Anyone can make a few decisions toward a goal, but a daily commitment requires serious motivation. The motivation can come from anywhere, and it is a good idea to surround yourself with positivity and motivation.

When someone makes a decision, constant feedback is a very good way to keep the train on the tracks. Surrounding yourself with other people on the same journey who can provide feedback will actually help you follow through with your goals.

Support in making the right decisions can come in two forms. Contingency management typically involves an outside agent who monitors behavior and delivers reinforcement when goals are met (e.g., Washington, Banna, & Gibson, 2014). Self-management typically involves observing and recording one's own behavior and can be used in conjunction with contingency management (Lynda Hayes).

When wanting to make a transformation, a lot of people hire some form of coach. Whether it is a personal trainer or a life coach, this may be a good avenue for beginners to pursue. We advocate exploring any and all routes that you can learn from. However, if you hire a trainer and just do what you're told to complete a transformation but do not learn why you are doing the things, it becomes difficult to sustain the new you. You have to become competent in making your own decision because contingency management is not going to hold your hand 24/7. At times you will be by yourself without your support system around you and you still need to make the right choices. If you do choose the path of outside help to accomplish your goals, the most important thing is to learn and internalize the meaning behind everything you are doing so that one day you can become self-sufficient—making you a stronger, better person!

"What you eat in private is what your wear in public."
~ Unknown Author

In order to strengthen decisions, you must increase your belief system. The question people often throw around is, "What would you do if you knew you could not fail?" If you knew beyond a shadow of a doubt that if you put your mind to something, you could accomplish it, there would be no excuse for not achieving your dreams. Why can we not think with this level of unwavering belief when it comes to our health and fitness?

Making the initial choice is often the easiest thing to do. We can all make a decision and set a goal to accomplish something. The factor that separates the achievers from the typical person is the follow through. When an achiever makes a decision, they tackle it knowing beyond a shadow of a doubt they will accomplish what they set out to accomplish. They know every day, no matter what gets thrown at them, they are going to continue taking steps toward their goals. When the initial decision is made, in their heads it's done. There is nothing left but to do it! When you make a decision, you have to couple that decision with the belief system that you can and will reach your goals.

Your belief system has to be built on solid rock. It has to be a foundation where even the mightiest of storms couldn't move it. Your beliefs have to be so strong in what you're trying to accomplish that no amount of setbacks or negativity will stop you. We do not live in a perfect world that caters to our every need. We live in the real world and have real problems. We are human and will stumble from time to time. But that belief system you have so deeply engrained into your psyche will get you back on track and keep you going.

Often at the first sign of trouble, people abandon the ship. Those are the people with no faith in their captain. In this analogy you are the captain of your life. Are you going to bail with the first sight of a rain cloud, or are you going to batten down the hatches and sail till you reach your destination?

Also, a big part of The Struggle is emotionally making decisions as mentioned earlier. One prime example of this is Karol and I both struggle with emotional eating. We associate food with pleasure, and it provides us a temporary escape from the cause of the underlying emotions we are trying to deal with.

Karol

"Emotional eating my way through the storm and for many years after is how I dealt with pain."

After Hurricane Katrina, my emotional eating was the worst ever. The emotional eating was my crutch; it numbed my pain at the realization of losing it all. It was my cigarette, my liquor and my Xanax all thrown into a bowl and topped with chocolate sauce, whipped cream, sprinkles and a cherry. It numbed every emotion I had and made the pain of losing it all just not hurt so badly. All the while I was hurting myself physically and mentally.

I truly ate my way through six months of the agony—the realization that my dreams and my life had changed dramatically due to Hurricane Katrina—and all I could do was find comfort in food. I don't drink or smoke anymore and did not want to take any anti-depressants, so I choose food to get me through. It tasted so good, but it was so detrimental to my health mentally and physically. I was on the biggest spiral down of my life and I knew one more Snickers bar would do the trick and make me feel better. I pass by the candy aisle today and flash back to ten years ago when I used to buy five to six candy bars a day and think this can't be as bad as a cigarette, can it? Sure it can. When I walked into the clinic and got my ass handed to me, literally from my doctor, I thought back to how my emotional eating, my bad choices, my lack of exercise, led me to 227 pounds. And, I knew food could not fix the pain. I knew I had to FIX it!

Exercise 3:

In chapter two you explored your past decision making. Now take time to write down the answers to these questions. What are the subconscious choices you regularly make without thinking that impacts the outcome of your life? What are the biggest influences on your decision-making process?

Chapter 4

Understanding the Commitment and Discipline

Robby

*I had to turn negativity in my life into something positive
and use it as fuel to achieve my goals.*

In the middle of my transformation I hit a low spot. The relationship I was in was at a very rocky and unstable point. I lost one job and had to start a new one where I was putting in a minimum of seventy hours per week. As we all know, when times get hard we often put our health on the back burner. I did just that. I spent all of my time at work or trying to mend my relationship. So in my head there was zero time left for my fitness goals and me.

I lost sight of what was important and I lost who I was. I was so focused on making everyone around me happy, I became miserable myself. In my head I did not have one positive thing to be thankful for (Stinkin Thinkin). I let a couple of negative circumstances destroy who I was. Even though I was at rock bottom, or so I thought, I knew I had to claw, fight and dig my way out of this hole.

The first thing I did was to rededicate myself to the gym. I would often go before work or during my lunch break, and if worst comes to worst, I would muster up the energy to go after a long twelve-hour workday. I made it a priority. While at work, the high point of my co-workers' days was what very unhealthy thing they were going to eat for lunch, whether it be fast food or the incredibly good authentic Asian restaurant right down the street. The constant barrage of temptation was hard for me because of my love for food.

For the first time in my life, I started meal prepping and making sure I had healthy meals and snacks packed with me at all times. I had to take a negative situation and make the best out of it. I had to focus on what was important to me and what made me happy even though emotionally I was in a terrible place. I believe that where there is a problem there is a solution.

When it seems like there is no hope and you cannot see the light at the end of the tunnel, your true character comes out. Your character can either rise to the challenge or succumb to the circumstances. It's all in your head. Those times are when you have to be stronger than the negatives and relentlessly pursue your goals. The most important lesson I learned through this process is you absolutely cannot make those around you happy when you are not even happy with yourself. If all you can think about is how rough your circumstances are and you play the role of the victim, how can others be happy to be around you? You have find that internal joy and let it shine, but it starts with you!

Now that you have cleared your head of the negative clutter and decided to make a drastic, positive change in your life, it is time to make the commitment.

Karol

"Commitment is relentlessly pursuing your goals even when the initial motivation wears off."

I Will Not Be Stopped
~ My Willpower Muscle

How badly do you want to achieve your goals? Is your goal something you just want to do or is it something you want to the point where no obstacle will stand in your way? As you read our stories, there are many highs and lows for both Robby and me. Many times we set goals and a lot of times, we sacrificed the goals for others or obstacles that got in the way. We allowed the derailment to happen then were frustrated about giving up on our goals.

There will ALWAYS be obstacles. There will always be big "detour" signs and roadblocks that will take you away from your goals. Things in your life will suck you in and take time and energy away from what is important to you. I do believe that when you set a goal, you have to factor in that someone or something just might and try to derail it. Well, not just might, it happens, and boy is that a Struggle.

Sometimes the possible derailing is intentional, whether it is your spouse not wanting you to get fit or your family not supporting you. Sometimes we just endure the everyday stresses in life—from working late and missing that spin class at the gym to the kids waking up late and you missing your Body Pump class. There always seem to be prime reasons why you can't stick to your goal. Obstacles in your way try and tug you mentally and physically from your goals. We say this several times, but this is when you have to set your goal and protect your goal. Like Under Armour, "You must protect this house."

You need to put guardrails around your goals and every time someone or something comes up and tries to pull you away from your goal, shut it down. Remember to ask whether that decision takes you CLOSER to your goal or farther away from your goal. Identify these factors as best as you can, put them on your vision board with a BIG X if you have to, and beware of the of the detours. Stay away from the roadblocks, stay on your course and protect your house.

One of the biggest weapons you have to protect you goals is your WHY. Your why is the reason you wanted make this change in the first place, the underlying reason you want to accomplish your goals. Your why is produced by your past and provides you with the motivation to transform your mind and body. The first thing you need to do is clearly define your WHY! Why do you want to make this change? What emotions and feelings led you to this decision? You have to have a deep down emotional attachment to why it is important to you for change.

> *"Your why has to be so strong that it makes you want to cry."*
> ~ *Hughie Smith.*

The Why lives deeply within you. This is where you will find it and once you own it, the decision to change is the easy part. The WHY you define will be your constant source of motivation when times get hard. When those detours pop up or when you yourself hit a road-block, the Why will get you through it. The WHY is what you look to when times get hard and negativity comes your way.

Your WHY gives you the fuel needed to pursue your goals, to push you out of bed thirty minutes early to go to the gym or on that early morning jog. The why will help you make better food choices when going out with your friends who love to celebrate with food and want to push food on you. You know doesn't align with your goals. The commitment and discipline to make drastic changes in your life is not easy, but nothing worth anything in life ever is. That is where your WHY plays a large part.

After you have fully come to grips with your WHY and understand the impact it is about to make in your life, you have to make it visible. You need to write down your why and put it somewhere you will see it every day. We put our WHY on the refrigerator, our vision boards, the bathroom mirror, above the home scale, in the office... Everywhere you need a source of reminding WHY it is so important for you make the right choices to accomplish your goals.

Commitment means doing what you know is right and what aligns with your goals even when the initial motivation wears off. Everyone wants to get better at something and can rally short-term motivation, but to truly accomplish goals, the motivation must persist through the struggles. Everyone has times where life tries to beat us down, but your commitment to your goals is what makes you get back up and start moving forward again.

"It's not whether you get knocked down. It's whether you get back up."
~ Vince Lombardi

Commitment and discipline become much easier when you truly have a burning desire to achieve your goals. When the desire to achieve your goals is deeply engrained into your heart, you do what you need to do to stay on the right path. If it is important to you, you will find a way.

You have to forget all the negatives and reasons you think you cannot accomplish your goals and push forward with an unwavering commitment until you succeed. The negativity of your past is like an anchor that can hold you back from moving toward your goals. The key is to understand your past it is just that—your past. With the power of choices and the impact the choices you make today have, you can rewrite the next chapter of your life. You have the ability and strength inside of you right now to stay focused and committed to your goals.

You need to see it, speak it and do it. You need to arm yourself with tools and motivation to help you succeed. You have to constantly feed the fire or it will simmer and die out. Understand clearly where you are and where you are going. A vision board is one helpful tool for visualizing what you want to achieve. Put positive quotes and pictures on it that can be a constant source of motivation. Write out your goals, put them on your board and read them every day.

You have to put you and your goals first in your thought process. As we talked about earlier, every choice is influenced by what you want the most. Is your desire to change more important to you than that pint of ice cream? By keeping your goals and your WHY in the forefront of your mind, you are able to stay more disciplined because you are thinking of the outcome of your choices versus just the here and now. The immediate gratification we are accustomed to takes a back seat to bigger, more important forms of gratification. The discipline needed to make a change goes hand in hand with willpower. The more you exercise it, the easier it becomes. Set small daily and weekly goals and outline how you will accomplish those goals. By setting short-term goals, you are not as overwhelmed with the whole process. As you win those battles to accomplish your goals, you gain a confidence and strength that starts to snowball making future goals seem easier to obtain.

Talk about your goals with others to build a support system and help you push to the next level or maintain discipline when times get hard. Find someone who can be a mentor to help you along this journey. Someone who has been there and knows the struggles you are going through is perfect. They have had the commitment and discipline to accomplish something you admire and can pour into you what has helped them on their journey. A mentor can often enlighten you to many of the mistakes they have made along their journey so you do not have to suffer the same setbacks.

In order to make time and stay focused on accomplishing your goals, you must prioritize what's important in your life. Ask yourself this—do my priorities align with my goals? Is my life aligned in a way that is conducive to my success? Through our many interviews asking people what they struggle with on their journey to achieve their goals, one reason came up time and time again. "I feel guilty for taking time away from my family."

Robby

Both of us are very close with our families and completely understand this struggle. I do not know where I would be without the love and support of my family. I come from a large Italian family that loves getting together over food and drinks. The guilt associated with taking time away from your family will be overtaken by the positive impact you have on them.

Please listen. It is ok to put you first, to make yourself a priority. We have to improve ourselves before we can help others. At times you may feel guilty about taking time away from your family or friends to accomplish these new goals. Sacrifices are part of any change in your life. One problem with sacrifice is the negative connotation most people associate with it. When you have a paradigm shift and realize that with sacrifice comes reward, you begin to understand the importance of making scarifies. In your head you have to associate sacrifices with rewards. If I give this up, I gain this. Most of the time the benefits are far more advantageous than the sacrifices you make.

In order to add something new, you must first take away. When you want something bad enough sacrifices are inevitable. Your lifestyle change is going to take sacrifices because you are in your current situation due to the choices you have made up to this point. You now have to sacrifice some things from your previous lifestyle to transform yourself to this new positive lifestyle. It really all boils down to—how badly do you want to accomplish your goals? Are your goals more important than the two hours of TV you watch every night? Are they more important than that donut at your favorite pastry shop? Is that thirty extra minutes of sleep more important than getting up and going for a twenty-minute walk?

Commitment and sacrifice go hand in hand—from something as small as sacrificing the taste of that donut for a protein shake to even as big as making your spouse watch your kids while you go and get your exercise. The single biggest thing you can do to make sacrifices not even feel like something you're giving up is remind yourself of your WHY. You are not sacrificing; instead you are gaining and improving. Think about how good it will feel to make that small sacrifice for a larger reward. The choice you have made to change your life and stay committed is a long-term goal and forgoes the immediate gratification of those perceived sacrifices. When you sacrifice what you want for everyone else, you end up becoming unhappy in the process. That brings everyone else around you down. Unhappiness and negativity are very contagious.

When making the decision to change and reprioritize your life, you still need balance. You have just made your mind up and committed yourself to accomplishing this new goal, which is going to bring about many positive changes. The one thing you cannot do is lose your balance. You cannot become so focused on changing your mind and body that the rest of the world around you comes crumbling down. You still need to spend time with your family and perform at your job. After all, bills don't pay themselves.

The balance is going to provide you stability through this transformation. If you spend all your time at the gym or running and neglect your spouse, how supportive do you think they will be of your goals? Of course the best-case scenario would be your family joins you in this journey, but that is not always the case. The change you are making in your life is yours and yours alone, but it also gives you the opportunity to show those around you it is possible. Keep in mind the transformation journey has to be enjoyable or you will give up. Find the balance and thus find the joy in your new commitment. You are on this journey to improve your life and bring you happiness.

You are now making a huge commitment that will drastically alter your life. You are doing this for yourself, but at the same time those around you will take notice. When people start noticing you change from the inside out, they will inevitably want to talk with you about it. The ensuing conversation is your opportunity to share your story and your WHY. When you have these conversations with people, they provide you with motivation to stay committed to your goals. Imagine the commitment level you will have when you now have others looking at you for a source of motivation and strength.

Remember that guilt you were feeling about taking time away from your family? Imagine how good it's going to feel to be the spark for your family to start living a healthier life. How good is it going to feel when you are motivating those around you to be healthy and possibly live longer?

My passion for helping others is paying off!

I have seen this in my own family. My entire family is being more active and making healthier food choices. My dad often jokingly tells me I am no fun to eat with anymore. We used to go eat all the buffets and buy all kinds of ice cream and stuff ourselves. He says this, but at the same time he's asking me what the healthiest type of oil to cook with is or what types of foods he should be eating. My mother is the same way. She is constantly asking me for healthy recipes or for advice on what healthy snacks she can bring with her to work.

Besides your family you can also be this way with your friends, co-workers, or really anyone you meet. A lot of research has been done that focuses on the influence peer reinforcement has on decisions and more importantly staying committed to those decisions. When people give you compliments on your progress or ask you what you have been doing to look so good, it encourages you to keep going and it makes those sacrifices easier.

Your life is constantly changing and you must adjust to the changes and maintain your priorities. Life never throws you strikes down the plate like a home run derby to better serve you. Curveballs are inevitable! We have to deal with these changes and roll with the punches. At times you will be so busy and stressed at work that finding the energy to go to the gym may seem impossible. We all have circumstances that come into our lives unexpectedly and test our commitment and fortitude. We all deal with stress, negative people, and deaths of those close to us, which can have deep emotional impacts in our lives. You may have just lost ten pounds and are feeling great about your accomplishment then all of the sudden your child falls and injures himself. Most parents' reaction to this would be to stay home and nurse their child back to health. It's a natural response. The problem comes in when we let that circumstance lead us away from our goals.

In this day and age, everyone has at one time used a GPS navigation system. The brilliant thing about GPS systems is the rerouting function. When you miss a turn or take the wrong exit, the GPS automatically adjusts your route and keeps you on track to your destination. We have to live our lives like a GPS system. We know what destination we are trying to reach and we know the straight shot route to get there. But what happens when we get knocked off track? We must not continue wandering around aimlessly hoping to find our way back on route. We must handle the curveball or setback in whatever form it may be and turn our eyes back to the destination. When using a GPS, you never know what road will be closed or if there is construction and you have to take a detour, but thanks the guidance system you are never lost. Use your internal GPS to give yourself focus and an unwavering sense of direction in your life.

Karol

Ready, Set, GOALLLLLL! How I kept my eye on the prize.

I use my bikini story from Key West to show you how this truly applies to setting goals. I am very goal oriented, and setting a goal with a date for me is crucial. It gives me something to work toward and gives me my daily motivation to work harder and reach my goals. I need smaller milestones as opposed to "I am going to lose fifty pounds in three months." Sometimes these larger goals are not achievable and not as specific.

So, when I found out about my sister's destination wedding, it was on. I set myself a goal to tone up and lose some more weight. My reward was to confidently, comfortably and fearlessly wear one bikini a day in Key West. The pressure was on, and I turned the pressure up on me, but being goal oriented, it worked for me. I added pictures on my vision board of Key West, I added pictures of fitness models wearing bikinis, and I added a recent picture of me. This way, I could see it visually and use my board as an anchor of motivation and inspiration to track my progress.

I added in extra cardio every day. Whether it be in the a.m. or p.m., I kicked it up a notch. I tracked my food and really paid attention to the small, hidden calories from creamer to an extra spoonful of peanut butter. I was very vigilant in my tracking, so I could really account for my actions to get me closer to my goal.

I tapped into my support system, my family and friends, when I felt like I needed a boost, and that always helped me. I posted my daily progress and promised myself I would post at least two to three pictures of me in my bikini at Key West. I made it my priority, I stayed focused and guess what, the world did not end because my priority was me. It was actually a better place for me.

So many of us feel so "guilty" to take time for us—an extra thirty minutes in the gym, cooking and prepping meals. It's OK to take time for you. You cannot be your best if YOU are not your best. I apply this to my time for me, gym time, and I know that time for me is more than physical. It is so mental for me. It gets me right and gives me the self-confidence I need. It nourishes my self-esteem and my soul, and to me, there is no better feeling. My priorities were making time for me, being accountable for me and working toward a healthier, fitter me, aligned with my goal.

I saw progress, week after week, which ALWAYS motivated me. Even the slightest, looser clothes, definition in my muscles, it all drove me. So, when it came time for Key West and the wedding, I was ready. I had reached my goal and it felt great. I sported my bikinis every day, feeling YES, Fearless, confident and strong. I took pictures and I looked at them. I felt great and to me, I looked great.

I worked hard in Key West to continue on my path, I got on a spinning bike at the gym every day for an hour, lifted weights, swam, and rode bicycles. Knowing I was indulging a bit on food, I upped my exercise and stayed the course. To reach this goal was one of my proudest times I had experienced in a long time. I just kept my actions in line with my goals and stayed focused on the prize.

One curveball that most of us face is negativity. The key to dealing with negativity is to identify the negatives that are a constant anchor in your life and get rid of them. You have to know what holds you back and challenge that negativity to make it positive. We have discussed that your reaction to outside influences must become a conscious thought process. How you react is a decision you make. We all have negative people in our lives who, because of their own insecurities, try and bring us down with them. Whenever they see us doing something positive in our lives, they feel the need to drag us back down to where they are. We all have our own struggles in life and often when people make negative comments about us, it is because they are struggling with something in their own lives. They are projecting their problems onto us to make themselves feel better. Remember that the next time you hear a negative comment.

Negativity can weigh you down more than a ton of bricks. It can and will break your spirits and kill your motivation, if you allow it to. Negativity affects us and everyone around us. It limits our potential to become what we desire, what we know is inside of us yearning to come out—to become something GREAT and live a healthy, fit lifestyle. Numerous medical studies have shown that negativity has a tangible effect on our health. Research shows that people who hold on to negativity cultivate negative energy, experience more stress and see health consequences. Negativity could even shorten the course of their lives as opposed those who choose to live positively.

Make the decision right now to rid yourself of negativity. When you make the decision to be positive and follow through on your decision, you will begin to encounter positive people and situations you never even knew existed. Someone who could drastically change the course of your life may have been there the whole time, but do to negativity you just could not see them. Do not let the mental anguish of negative people affect YOU, mentally or physically.

You can take several steps right now to rid yourself of negative energy and become positive. Create your Mental Shield. It is easier said than done to rid yourself of all of the negatives in your life. After all, you may have a deep connection with some of them. If it is someone close to you, talk with them about this new direction in your life. Open communication is the key. Think of your mental shield as a deflector, something to keep the negative out and only allow the positive to flow in.

Karol's Shield of Armor

Try this to create your armor. I call it my Shield of Positivity. I literally get dressed in the morning and mentally put my shield of positivity on. I prepare myself for the day with the notion that yes, there will be negative people and situations that will try and attack my shield, but my positivity is stronger and it will persevere anything thrown at it. Many people thrive on being negative. It feeds their pessimistic outlook on life. They try to bring others down with them and the more people to share in their misery the better. If you are going to do something positive in your life, you can't be around this type of people because negativity is contagious. You do not want to participate and be brought down from the negativity and allow yourself to be distracted from your goals.

Change the way you talk to yourself. We all go through the day having a constant dialogue with ourselves that influences every choice we make. Negativity like a cancer can start small inside of you, and if you are not careful it will consume your entire world. It is very damaging to your self-image and changing this thought process takes a lot of positive self-talk. The next time you have negative thoughts, write them down, reflect on them and rephrase them, changing the cant's to can and the won't to will. Visually it will help you push through. Sometimes we are our own worst critics. We are the ones who focus on our own negative thoughts. Changing your self-talk is one of the most powerful things YOU can control.

You have to find your own way of dealing with negativity because you simply cannot just avoid it at all times.

Robby

I use doubt to fuel my competitive spirit.

Karol and I both channel negativity to fuel our goals. I love it when someone tells me, "You'll never have that. You'll never be able to look like that." All that does is add fuel to my fire. I take that as a challenge and I rather enjoy proving people wrong. Sometimes we have the ability to avoid certain negatives in our lives. If you know that watching all the food porn on TV is going to create internal negativity, don't surround yourself by it. Avoid the negatives you know you will come across as much as you can until you are strong enough not to give in. Your WHY will also help you combat negativity. The next time you feel negativity in your life rewrite out your why and remember how important it is to you.

Food reinforcement is often a problem that many of us deal with. Everything we do in life we associate with food. When we celebrate the accomplishments in our lives, it generally revolves around food and drinks. When was the last time all of your family or friends were together when the focal point was not of food? I told you, I come from a large Italian family that loves eating. When I was growing up oftentimes my grandmother would spend a week preparing food for a get together. I still can hear my mom and my aunts planning who was bringing what dish. It is a part of our culture and always has been. We are not saying don't enjoy these times and these incredible meals. Just don't let them derail you from you goals. Remember you have to find your balance.

Just like we talked about the power or choices and gaining control of our thought processes, we have to realign this area with our goals as well. You have to find new ways to reinforce your accomplishments without something that is going to set you back. If you have just accomplished a goal or had something special happen in your life, look for a more positive way to reward yourself. You can buy a new pair of skinny jeans, go relax by the pool or get a massage as your new reward system. Find positive ways to reinforce your behaviors that will help you accomplish your goals.

The level of motivation we have to accomplish our goals is like a roller coaster ride. Some days we have the motivation to conquer the world and other days we do not even have enough to get out of bed much less eat healthy and workout. These are just the ebbs and flows of life.

In order for your commitment and discipline to stand the struggles of life, you must find a source of constant motivation. Motivation, like willpower, is also a limited resource, which is why you need to find what motivates you. Your source of constant motivation (your **WHY**) needs to be internal but can also come from external resources. Your Why has to be the most important reason why you want to change your life for the better, but we all get weak at times and need external motivation to get us through those struggles. Whether it is a workout buddy or your favorite fitness magazine, find that motivation that will get you closer to your goal.

Even as strong as we all are, we need to surround ourselves with sources of inspiration and motivation. With the rise of social media and Internet-based communities, there is never a lack of inspirational personalities and sources of motivation at your fingertips. With just a few clicks, you can have access to that source of motivation you need to pick you back up and get you back on track. From blogs to You-Tube personalities and Instagram, you can find a source or individual you identify with who understands what you're battling and going through.

What I Use to Stay Motivated

I draw most of my external motivation from YouTube. I keep up with my favorite YouTube fitness personalities and watch as they grow, stay committed, face the same struggles I do, and eventually conquer their goals. They may not be right here with me to help with food choices or push me through a workout, but after seeing others like me persevere through the hard times to accomplish great things, it give me the strength to do it myself. So to all the YouTube Fitness Vloggers, keep up the hard work and know that what you are doing is helping others in ways you never imagined.

There are many aspects to staying committed and disciplined with your transformation, but the most important thing is to keep moving forward. There will be times when you have to readjust your priorities and make sacrifices you never thought you would. You will take yourself out of your comfort zone. You have to remind yourself that achieving your goals is the reward you are searching for. You have three choices associated with your goal—give up, give in or give it everything you got. Don't let life change your goals because achieving your goals will change your life.

"Do not settle for less than exactly what you want. Your heart's desires are there for a reason, chase them. Pursue relentlessly, do not lose sight of your goals, they are your very reason for being."
~ Franki Durbin

Exercise 4:
Visualize what success looks like to you. Now write down your vision and all the reasons why it is important for you to achieve that goal. How badly do you want it? Also, write down the potential hurdles you may face so you can recognize them and not let them slow you down on your journey.

Chapter 5

Gaining the Knowledge

Robby

Discovering the Power of Self-Education

When I first started my transformation, I had no idea what I was doing. I just knew what I wanted to accomplish. I knew I was tired of the old me inside and out, and I had to decide what I wanted. Until that decision I had always been the type of person who just went with the flow, and since college athletics was such a huge part of my life, it seemed like I was just always doing what I was told to do.

My transformation was the first time in my life I was 100% in control. I now needed a new skill set to accompany my new direction. I knew how to be this massive football player, but that is not what made me happy. I thoroughly enjoyed my time playing college football and have zero regrets, but in order to achieve this new goal, I had to embrace change. At that time I started asking myself, "Well, what do I do now? How do I do this? What do I eat? How do I train?"

All these thoughts were overwhelming, but I went on a personal knowledge crusade! I started researching, reading articles, talking to the fit people I saw in the gym, watching videos, just anything and everything I could get my hands on to increase my knowledge. I discovered an insatiable appetite for knowledge. I knew the best route for me to accomplish my goals was to actually learn how to do it and understand the why behind it.

You have often heard that knowledge is a weapon. Well it could not be truer in the world of health and fitness. I wanted to arm myself with every available resource I could. I knew making such a drastic change in my life would be an everyday battle, and who wants to go into battle with their hands tied behind their back?

Another part of my education process was to learn my own body. I had to learn how my body reacted to certain foods and which style of training my body best responded to. Individuals are genetically different and their bodies respond and metabolize food differently. What is good for me and provides me with the greatest amount of sustained fuel for my workouts may cause you to have an energy crash. I challenge you to not only gain external knowledge but also pay attention and learn from your body.

When we make something a priority in our lives, we give it precedence. Many people have the motivation to lose weight but simply lack the knowledge. As we were conducting interviews with numerous people, one large reason we continually heard as to why people never began their new healthy lifestyle was they didn't know where to start. They had the internal desire to change but simply never started because they lacked the knowledge of how to do it. They became completely overwhelmed to the point of quitting before they ever took the first step.

In chapter three we discussed how this seemingly complicated decision is actually very simple—To be Healthy or Not. Once you make the decision, you just have to start moving forward. You made the decision to better yourself and your life, but now you have to arm yourself with the weapons to win the battle.

You can be the best racecar driver in the world with the best racing fuel ever engineered, but unless you are in the right car you simply cannot win. It takes everything working together synergistically. You are the driver. Your WHY and commitment are your fuel. Your knowledge is the car that will ensure victory. Knowledge related to your new health and fitness lifestyle is crucial for your success. You simply cannot just know what to do. You need to understand why you are doing it. Why is this better for me than that? Why are we doing this exercise over that one? Understanding the why behind the knowledge you gain is equally important.

Today, with technology and information at our fingertips, the opportunity to gain knowledge is more accessible than ever. Print media has gone digital and is accessible from any device with an Internet connection. You can sign up for e-mails, newsletters from health and fitness pages, and receive information on health, nutrition and fitness. From blogs to articles posted daily on social media, the knowledge is attainable if you want it. We both follow a number of websites and fitness personalities to garner the knowledge. The resources are all around you and in abundance from social media to actual self-help groups. Meal plans, exercise plans, and all aspects of your new lifestyle are now easy to find. It is up to you to gain the knowledge and educate yourself. The knowledge you can equip yourself with is amazing!

If this new journey you are about to embark upon is important in your life, you will become hungry for knowledge. You should have an appetite for knowledge because knowledge is your power. The ability to gain knowledge and educate yourself from the experts in the fitness and health industry will only help you get closer to achieving your goal. Feed that knowledge appetite by finding some good resources to learn from or even find meetings and groups where you can gain the knowledge.

There is a wealth of knowledge to tap into and most is free. Examples are YouTube, Twitter, Facebook Fitness Websites. Find fitness professionals online that you identify with and follow them. Find a personality that engages you and learn from their success and their struggles. We have both learned so much from following these fitness professionals, nutritionists, dieticians, and medical experts via social media and beyond. We are not proponents of everyone reinventing the wheel. Use the resources available and apply them in your own life. If you need a new healthy snack or a new healthy recipe to prepare for your family, go find it.

You have to educate yourself. No one is going to put the knowledge in your head if you don't want it there, so that means you must take action. And the easiest part about it is that the knowledge is all literally right at your fingertips.

Karol

Some other great resources to tap in are audio books. I enjoy listening to audio books, and I read as many fitness magazines as I can, from Clean Eating to Oxygen to Yoga. I read and arm myself with the knowledge I need to in order stay the course, and you can do this too.

Growing up, my parents shared this resource with me. They actually instilled it in me to eat healthy, as my mother was a nurse. We ate very clean meals and my dad and mom, both being extremely physically active, got me involved in sports and activities at a very young age. That was the easy part. Now, all grown up and hungry for knowledge as to how I can get myself healthier, fitter, and leaner, I have to educate myself and tap into all the resources I can.

If you want to win the race, you must put the right fuel in your car! Knowledge is fuel for your journey. By arming yourself with the facts about eating healthy and exercising, you can DO THIS!

We talked about finding knowledge in books, articles, and web sites but other great resources are family and friends, a self-help group, health professionals, health clubs, and forums about health and fitness. Tap into any resource you can via work, friends, family and most importantly, find dependable resources. Educate yourself on not only the physical, workout side but also the food and the nutrition sides as well.

Then you are going to have to dig deeper, look into yourself and ask yourself, why you're doing what you're doing. This was the hardest thing for me to face, besides the scale and the mirror. To truly understand why…do you use food as an emotional crutch? And where do you gain the knowledge to address that action and learn how to control it?

Don't be afraid to ask for knowledge. Find someone you aspire to be like and just have a conversation with them. Ask about their motivations, where they find discipline, and how they achieved their goals. People who have transformed themselves enjoy sharing their journey and are very proud of their accomplishments. They will share with you instantly, so take their knowledge and apply it to your life.

The why is what gets you started, but the how is your key to continued success. A journey to health is not a sprint. It is a lifelong journey. Many people yo-yo diet because they don't understand what they are doing and why they are doing it. Many people think they know how to lose weight, and they might find temporary success, but lack the knowledge of the healthiest way to do it for the long run.

One of the first places we encourage you to learn from is your past. We all can look back and say, if I knew this, I would have not done this. If you are like most people, including both of us, the best educational experiences of your life have been lessons you learned the hard way. Looking back at our pasts we can see that without even knowing we were constantly learning and evolving from our own experiences. After all, your past has made you who you are today—good or bad. The good news is your past mistakes are meant to guide you not define you. We must look at choices we have made to learn from them and not make them again in the future.

"Those who do not learn from history are doomed to repeat it."
~ George Santayana

At times in your past when you have failed to succeed, it may have been due to not knowing what you needed in order to achieve your goals. Did you have the resources to gain the knowledge? If you didn't, why not? Now that you understand the importance, educate yourself with the knowledge that will help you achieve your goals.

Robby

I used trial and error to learn what works best for my body.

As you progress on your new journey, you will be learning a lot of information from outside sources. But to really understand how to apply that knowledge, you must learn your own body. We are proponents of trial and error within reason. I know I have tried every diet under the sun. Every new piece of research that came out, I would latch on to it and think, "This is the missing link I have been searching for!"

Through trying countless diets, I paid close attention to how much my body reacts to certain types of food and what effect the timing of certain foods has on my body. Everyone's body will react differently to variables and stimuli. You may only require twenty minutes of activity per day to lose weight while the person next to you on the same exact diet has to spend forty-five minutes. The knowledge of how your body functions is very powerful. When you gain knowledge into how your body works, what food is good to eat, when it is prime time to eat certain things, and what other nutrients your body needs, this will all help you make better choices. If you don't know, how can you really make good choices?

Complete self-education takes you back to school to study up on what is going to help you make better choices—the right choices this time. The difference is you no longer have to ask the teacher why you need this class. When am I going to use this again? You will use it every day in every choice you make to become the healthiest version of you.

Karol

Going The Distance—Life is a Marathon, Not a Sprint
My Weight Watchers Journey

Knowledge will help you learn to make the right choices. I found this most helpful when I started learning more about food and nutrition, what I need to fuel my body, what I need to lean my body out, and what I need to put in my body to perform at its best. Also, learning what foods work for me—superfoods and greens—help me make better choices, which lead to me reaching my goals.

Yearning for knowledge to apply to my life led me to Weight Watchers. That and I literally hated looking at myself in pictures. I had such a great smile, but I was dying inside and was so overwhelmed with my weight and my emotional eating to ease the stresses of my world. I love fitness. That never swayed and I knew I still had good muscle mass and muscle memory, but I couldn't remember the last time I had worked out and eaten healthy.

So, in 2003 I joined Weight Watchers with my friend Sylvia to learn, re-educate myself and gain the knowledge of what my body needs not wants. I needed to gain the knowledge of eating right, eating the right portions, and tracking my progress coupled with exercise. And, at Weight Watchers, the magic happened for me. I had the most amazing leader, Pam Davis, and just as important, I had a Sunday morning (yes, I called it my church) group of people who were consistent with attending a real self-help group in more ways than weight loss.

Every week, we received a new booklet on the topic of the week, success stories from other members, great, easy recipes along with tips to get us going. The topic of the week was always relatable. It was as though they'd lived in my head and pulled out the topic from me every week. I could so relate. I could so empathize with what I was going through as well as the others in the room.

Every week, Pam would lead our class as we discussed the topic and always asked for input and feedback on the topic. I would feverishly write down what she had written down along with other information I felt was applicable to me, which was ALL of it. I was amazed at how much we would cover in an hour. It was very raw at times, a lot of us breaking down. Yes, I cried many tears of joy and sadness, accepting responsibilities for my actions, which made me the person I had become. Every week, I could gain knowledge on how I could own it, improve me, educate myself, and gain the knowledge I needed to change the course of my life. Did I tell you I was hard headed? Yep, it took quite some time, a few years actually of staying on track, going to my meetings and therapy combined to finally get it right, FOR GOOD, for it to STICK. As my gymnastics coach would say, "Stick it!"

I would lose thirty, gain forty back over time. I would stop going to the meetings and therefore was not getting the knowledge and support I needed to make this change and to understand why I emotionally eat, my triggers, and what was I trying to drown. But, in 2008—yes, five years after I joined, due to my wellness visit for my work—I got it, my magic moment, my epiphany.

I had to apply the knowledge and believe in what I now know to be the best two years of my life as far as gaining knowledge to change me for good, for once and for ALL. And, I did, I applied all the knowledge I had gained from going to the classes, going to boot camp to exercise again, gaining knowledge from my trainer Luke and finally applying it to ME, Karol. And guess what? I was finally seeing results, the results that only come when you apply what you have learned and stay the course.

I attended class every Sunday. I wrote down my notes, and I would read them often during the week. I got the e-mails, got support from my family and friends, but most importantly what I needed to arm myself with was knowledge. With it came a lot of tough questions that WW does identify and speak about often. They discuss triggers as to why you eat—emotional eating and what that does to you, mentally and physically. And yes, just like you, I had to ask myself the hard questions. Why? Why am I doing this to myself? What emotionally is wrong that I have to eat to emotionally take the pain away? And what are the triggers that cause me to emotionally eat?

I had so many emotions that I never addressed after Hurricane Katrina and losing everything—so much heartache, pain, so much sadness inside of me. I was almost in disbelief that my life changed that quickly, and the only thing that made the pain and heartache go away was food. Yep, some heavy, heavy questions, but I knew I had to answer them in order to truly change the course of my life.

As hard at is was, it was my necessary evil because the 3 Musketeers were not telling me what I needed to hear and address—my emotions. I think of this process as the onion process. I had to literally, mentally peel back years of grief, heartache and humiliation with the outcome from Hurricane Katrina that washed away my relationship and my business. I just continued to eat through the pain and devastation I had amassed. Even though I had moved on to a new career for Gary and me, it was so emotional, and the hurt of losing our business and us in one swoop, was my tipping point.

I came to realize during this time that I needed to address my feelings and my emotions. I did, and I not only did I let it out at WW classes, but I went to a therapist who helped me peel back my feelings and emotions and helped me deal with them one layer at a time. She made me realize that Katrina was not my fault. Losing my business from Katrina did not make me a failure like I thought I was, and that my heart would heal in time.

She made me address these emotions and then go work out after we had a session. It was so raw, but I would leave it at the gym, one layer at a time. After a while, I started to ease up on myself and realize that I can't carry the guilt of a natural disaster on my shoulders, but I can carry weights on my shoulders to get stronger.

I knew this time I had the knowledge to fall back on. I was equipped with the tools I needed to address my emotional eating, my stress eating and change my habits to good, healthy habits. I learned to use exercise as a great stress reliever. I added in cardio after a long day at the office or made it the first thing in the morning to relieve my stress of work.

I was committed to my food diary, and I wrote down all the food I consumed along with the calories, fat, etc. This way I could really see what I was putting in my body. Knowledge...I had it. I had gained so much knowledge from my WW classes by listening, learning and applying the knowledge to me. And, yes, I made major headway.

In two years, I had lost one hundred pounds. What an accomplishment! I had laid my foundation, my knowledge, coupled with my willpower and my commitment to me. It yielded a NEW me, a fixed me. I was not broken anymore, and I was not using food as my drug to numb the pain and the stress. Quite the opposite, I was using it to fuel my body to perform at its best. I felt great, like a thousand pounds had been lifted off my shoulders because I had the knowledge to change me.

We say this again and again, and here it goes again—the one hundred pounds came off by eating right and exercising. No special diet magic or skinny pill. I just strapped on the knowledge and applied it. I changed the way I thought and reacted, and because of this, I made better choices to reach my goal. In 2010, I reached my goal, and I submitted my story to Weight Watchers to be selected as Role Model of the Year. And I was! I received my letter in May 2010 from WW corporate that I had been selected, and I was ESTATIC. I now could share my story of gaining knowledge, applying it my everyday life and changing the course of my life for the better.

Finally, inside and OUT, I was on top of the world. I ran a half marathon that February—13.1 miles—and in May, I finally reached my weight goal and was selected as a Role Model. I knew my moment had come, and I knew I had a story to share to motivate others. I still take such pride in sharing my Role Model of the Year story and my WW journey with anyone I can.

I continue use many techniques I learned from WW along with the knowledge I gained from attending class. I am so very grateful to my friend Sylvia who convinced me to join with her, everyone in class, and the most amazing instructor ever. Thank you, Pam, for your unwavering support you gave everyone. During the good weeks and bad weeks, you were always there. Thank you for your guidance and your passion to help others.

Robby

"Knowledge without ambition is like a bird without wings"
~ Salvador Dali

Above is one of my favorite quotes. This truly speaks to how important it is to implement your new knowledge on your journey. Learning is a never-ending process that you must continue throughout your transformation. You have to use that knowledge as a weapon to attack your goals. Even if you completely understood the biomechanics and chemistry of the best diet in the world, if you do not implement the principles of the diet into your life, how do you expect to find success?

Your WHY will spark the fire, and your motivation and knowledge will fuel the fire. But you have to constantly add fuel or the fire will burn out. You will use your education combined with your WHY as a shield to protect yourself from what we all know as The Struggle. During times when you have to make decisions, you now have equipped yourself with the knowledge to avoid pitfalls. Your knowledge is a shield you wear every day to not only guard you but to give you strength in your choices. When you know what foods will do to your body and understand the impacts of living an active lifestyle, you begin to make choices with conviction. I promise knowing that piece of chocolate cake for dessert has 350 calories and will take you forty-five minutes on the treadmill to burn off will play a role in your decision making.

You are the one making the decision to self-educate, but another influence on your education that few people think about is your surroundings. You are a product of those surrounding you. More precisely you are the product of the five closest friends/family members in your life. You have to make the decision to purposely surround yourself with like-minded individuals who are goal oriented and have the same passion you do for a healthy, fit life! The benefits of surrounding yourself with like-minded people are numerous. They become a great source of motivation and knowledge. It also is a great opportunity to share your successes and setbacks and gain motivation from your support system. You cannot go on this journey alone. It's not fun and you need the support to get you through the tough times and celebrate your successes.

I firmly believe you are the product of those surrounding you.

Some of the fastest progress I have made in my journey has been when I have surrounded myself with those I aspire to be like. I am a huge advocate of including people in your life who will challenge you and make you better. Find someone you can just tell is leading a healthy lifestyle and being positive, and find ways to include them in your life. The more you are around challenging people, the more you'll be forced to grow to keep up.

I very rarely work out with a workout partner because normally that's my "me time." I put my music on, get lost in the workout and totally forget the world. When you do see me working out with someone, it is for one of two reasons. Either someone has approached me to better themselves, or I have found someone who can really push me to test my limits. As with most people time is my most precious limited commodity. I simply do not have time to surround myself with people who aren't one of those two types. When you are in the company of others who understand your struggles, who understand what you have been through, it allows you to more freely open up and express your own thoughts and feelings.

Karol

Where I Find My Support

Look at my story from Weight Watchers. This is a great example of where I found my support. And when I needed more, I looked to my closest friends. I had a co-worker, Jody. Around the same time I started getting serious about my decision to change my life for a healthy, fit life, she had committed to make a change to be healthier and fitter too.

I'll never forget, I asked Jody over for Thanksgiving one year as she was from California and my mom and I could not bear her being alone for Thanksgiving. It was 2008, and I look at that picture today and don't even recognize either one of us. Jody and I worked in the same department and had a small lunch area with one table and two chairs. But that's all we needed to bond. We had each other and great conversation.

We started eating lunch together, just chatting, quickly to realize we BOTH had made a big commitment to get HEALTY and FIT. So, we were each other's work buddies, support systems. We brought our lunch every day and would take our lunch breaks together to talk about our struggles and successes. We would bring our fitness magazines and talk about motivation stories from the mags, new fitness routines, and new recipes, which we tried a lot because Jody loved to cook. So, she was always cooking up something yummy. I preferred for Whole Foods to cook for me, so we did quite a bit of shopping together, learning a lot about nutrition, food and what healthy options there are to substitute the fat, yummy tasting stuff. She joined the gym, and then got a trainer.

I was so proud of her. We began to spend time out of work together, as we both loved music and festivals. We would walk in our city park and just chat. She made my journey feel effortless at times because we were both there for each other. We both made huge strides the next two years, continuing and staying committed to our healthy choices. She was my anchor, my support system, and today she is back home in California and has kept her weight off, enjoying her active lifestyle. That too makes me very happy knowing we BOTH made a commitment and kept it because of our support for each other. Thank you, Jody, for always being there for ME!

By sharing your story, your struggles and your progress with others, it will not only inspire and motivate them, but in return they can give you insight to the things they have learned on their journeys.

Remember, in order to grow you have to be in a constant state of learning.

Even for introverts, plenty of opportunities exist to surround yourself with other positive, like-minded individuals such as work out classes, support groups, work out partners, and any collection of people who share your goals and aspirations. The resources at your fingertips allow you to sit by yourself and gain the knowledge or be a part of a bigger movement. Whether it be a self-help group or a group class at the gym, find your support system and don't let go!

Also, remember the importance of getting rid of all the negativity in your life. All the knowledge in the world will slip through your fingers if you don't rid yourself of the negatives in your life NOW!!

Surround yourself with positive people, your "reinforcement shield." Since we become those most often surrounding us, you simply cannot continue your growth and education around negative influences.

If a circle of friends is full of negativity, energy-suckers, you will emulate that exact behavior and become just like them. These actions will not help you stay on course for a better, healthier, fitter lifestyle. It is very difficult to become more positive when the people around you—that circle of friends, co-workers, and even family sometimes— are constantly bringing you down.

As you make the change to become more positive, you will find that your existing friends will either appreciate the new, positive you or they will become resistant to your positive changes. Change is scary any way you look at it. People will come and go from your life as we all evolve and change. One of the toughest decisions you will ever make in life is distancing yourself from those who are close to you that are bringing you down. Part of this new you, the transformation you are going through, is to become a stronger, more positive you. When you do you accomplish your goals, you want to be a source of inspiration to others. No one wants to follow a negative Nancy.

Aspire to be a positive role model to others. If someone truly is your friend and a supporter of your goals, they are going to make you a better person. So, seek out these people, the ones who offer positive reinforcement, motivation and inspiration even if it takes you out of your circle of friends. You have to chart the positive course, and cutting out the negative people is a giant leap toward your goal.

Negative thoughts can be overwhelming and challenging to navigate. A lot of negativity brings on a "freak out" mode, as I call it. This is an emotional response out of our own fears and insecurities. It is especially impactful when tied to a relationship or person concerning the future unknown. The overwhelming feeling of negativity is debilitating and can literally rip apart all of your efforts to become positive. Negativity snowballs into more worry, more stress, more freak-outs and to me, more emotional eating.

You have to turn the negative stress into positive action today. The next time you are in freak-out mode, take a step back, and with your eyes closed, BREATHE, recompose yourself to not think emotionally but rather logically. Take yourself out of the situation emotionally. Don't allow any of this to cause any triggers that would drive you to making emotionally charged decisions or react in a negative way.

I Learned to Overcome My Emotional Eating

This was my biggest downfall, as the freak-outs gave me a green light to emotionally eat to ease my stress and my emotions. I have since learned how to deal with my freak-outs and not allow them to drive me to eat. Once you are calm enough and you are thinking rationally, take out pen and write down a few solutions to begin solving the problem without food. Taking yourself out of the current emotionally charged, negative train of thought by moving into the action-oriented positive will help you solve more problems rationally and, yes, without food. It will allow you to always live in positive state.

Self-discovery and education are vital toward your success. Everything from learning about exercise and nutrition to, more importantly, learning yourself will give you the strength to become the master of your emotions, reactions and decisions. You will understand why your body reacts the way it does to nutrition and exercise and even why you are having certain thoughts. If the journey to become the new you starts in your head, your body will reap the benefits. Arm yourself with knowledge today to have the future you want and deserve.

Exercise 5:

Write down some of the areas in your life where you need to learn more to progress toward your goals. What is one habit you are going to implement in your life to ensure you are in a state of constant learning? Why is it important to you to implement all of your newfound knowledge?

Chapter 6

Go

"Even the journey of a thousand miles starts with a single step."
~ Lao Tzu

Karol

The body achieves what the mind believes.
How I went the distance—all 13.1 miles.

Did you know that less than 1% of the world ever runs a Marathon? I never thought I would be part of that number. Growing up, I ran track because I was fast. I was not a runner per say, but I did participate in track and field growing up. Later in life, my sisters ran, so every now and then I would run with them. But it was not my exercise of choice. I much preferred being in the gym.

In 2010 all of that changed for me. I had a friend, Torie, who encouraged me to start walking with her and soon enough, I would run a little, walk a little, run a little, walk a little, then, run more and walk less. Before I knew it, I was running the whole way (yes, with a few breaks in between).

In the fall of 2009, the New Orleans Saints were winning and the excitement was in the air. I found my motivation from the Drew Brees' Huddle Talk and from his slogan, Finish Strong. I thought if these guys can dig deep, find their motivation and finish strong every time, so can I! So, Torie and I signed up for a 5K race, my first run. Yes, I was going to run it.

It was on the levee on the river, and I will never forget that morning. It was freezing and windy, super windy, but when they said go, I turned up my music and started running. Running is such a mind game, and as I was running, I had a lot of time to reflect on where I was in my life with my emotional eating and weight.

It was such a proud moment for me. I was running in a 5K race! I had focused on a goal and I was going to Finish Strong today. And I did. I was probably last in the running category, but that was so insignificant for me. What was important was that I set my goal, went for it and crushed it. Yes, I went the distance. Well, the running bug bit me after that and I decided I wanted to run the Rock N Roll Half Marathon in February in New Orleans—13.1 miles. That was a pretty aggressive goal to go from not running to a 5K to running a half a marathon, but that was my new goal. And yes, I was going to crush it!

So, Torie and I signed up for another race closer to the Rock N Roll, a 10K race this time. It was sure to get me ready for my 13.1 mile run. There were two jogging routes, one a shorter route and one the 10K route. So, off I went wearing my black and gold. I had a Huddle Talk from Drew Brees on my IPod, so I would play it before I ran. Then I would crank up the rock and roll and off I went.

I followed the pack because I was not a fast runner but more a consistent jogger. I got lost in the music and so inspired by so many people running, mostly past me, but we were all going in the same direction—a fit lifestyle and crossing the finish line. Well, somewhere along the path, I made a turn thinking this was the route for the longer run and I got lost. We were running through a pretty big industrial business park in the city, so I thought, hmmmm, I will run into the runners somewhere. I kept running. I had water with me so, I would stop have a drink then run on.

Well, I did this for what seemed like forever and I did not see one person. I knew then I was not only lost but had to run my way back to the route or at least the finish line. I finally ran into the trailing pack of walkers almost an hour later minutes later. It was the walkers. The runners had all crossed the finish line a long time ago. So, I peeled off and ran the other route that I thought was for runners and crossed the finish line.

Meantime, my friend Torie, the walker, was waiting for me. She said she and her friend Eddie were worried because almost everyone had finished but not me. I looked at my watch and it showed I had run 10 miles that morning, quite a bit more than 10K, which is 6.2 miles. I felt fearless. I could not believe I ran that far.

Just as we were getting our bags, a runner walked up to me and said, "You know, you cheated. I saw you cut the last block, and you did not finish the course." She was pretty upset about it. Little did she know I literally ran in circles and ran circles around her that morning. And yes, I am quite a passionate pepper, so, I firmly let her have it. I told her this was my second race and not only did I finish the course, I ran an extra four miles, so really she needed to be proud of me for running ten miles and that I finished strong. Yes, I did have some other strong words for her, sending her off with the fact that I ran circles around her.

Then, the big Day, February 2010, The Rock N Roll Half Marathon. Torie and Eddie were walking it, so they were in a different zone than me for the race. This was the Super Bowl of marathons and yes the Saints were going to the Super Bowl. So all the motivation I gathered from my home team I was taking on the race with me. It was in New Orleans, through some of my favorite places in my city, so I was excited to be a local running this race with the motivation at my back, pushing me to run. Don't stop. Go the distance.

There were over twenty-five thousand people signed up, and this was such a new world to me—so many people, so strong, so fit, so focused. I started to feel a little overwhelmed as these runners were serious runners and I was just a beginner. But, I took my headphones, turned on the Huddle speech and claimed my moment. I was ready, I was physically ready to run 13.1 miles and my willpower, my motivation, and my determination fueled my race. When the race gun went off, so did we.

A sea of people were literally everywhere, and I felt like I was in the desert running in a stampede with thousands of animals. You had to be quick. I finally found my pace, turned my music up and just ran, I took in the most beautiful sights of New Orleans and really appreciated being a part of such a big movement. I had to stop at mile nine to use the restroom, but after I waited twenty minutes and was no closer, I started running again and did not want to slow down or stop.

My parents, my sister Kim and my friend Jody were all on the route, cheering me on. I slowed down long enough to take a picture with my mom and dad and am so glad I did. They have been there for me in every aspect of my life and have been my biggest supporters for my weight journey. This time, they knew that with my willpower and my focus on my goals, I was going to succeed. I had changed my habits, and I had changed my life to ensure I would live a healthy, fit life, just like them. That moment when my mom and dad literally saw me and started cheering me on will stay with me forever. They were so proud and I was so proud to know that I did it with their help and that of MANY others.

I finished the race in about three hours—not the fastest but not the slowest. I got my medal, took a picture with my medal, found my friends at the post party and had a big cry of joy for myself. I felt like Rocky. I was on top of the world. I just ran a marathon and finished strong. That year, the Saints did the same. They won the Super Bowl. They finished strong and took home the Championship, and so did I. It goes to show you that one step, one good choice, one goal will get YOU to the finish line.

My marathon is not over by any means. I go the distance every day in making my healthy choices in fitness and exercise. And, when I struggle, I take my medal and rub it, knowing that I went the distance!

I put the emphasis on action, used all my motivation, set a goal and accomplished it. GO is what will move you in the direction you want to accomplish your goals. GO, get active, start eating right, making healthier choices and get moving. You will see results if you take action.

It's time to take action. Now that your why is deeply engrained into every aspect of your life and you have a deep burning desire to transform your life, the only thing left is to do it. You have removed all the excuses and reasons stopping you. Now is the time to have a laser beam of focus on what your heart truly desires. Up until this point in the book, we have given you all the necessary tools to equip you for your new lifestyle. Armed with the motivation and knowledge, it is now time to just do it.

You can have the best diet plan and the top personal trainer in the world, but if you fail to apply yourself, you will never succeed. You can gain access to all you need to accomplish your goals at your fingertips, but the main factor in this equation is YOU. You are the X variable and the most important one. Only you can take that first step and then put one foot in front of the other toward your goals. The only thing stopping you from becoming who you want to be is you. You 100% own this journey, and no one is going to do it for you. I wish someone would go run for me to burn my calories, but that simply work. I know that I alone am the only one who can change myself. I have the power, strength and desire to do it.

GO, Take Action, and envision the NEW YOU—a healthier and happier version of yourself!

We have all heard the classic clichés. NOW is the time. Life is short. Quit procrastinating. We are only on this earth for a very short time. We have heard these a million times, but time is our most precious commodity and we only have so much of it. Every passing minute is an opportunity lost for change. We cannot get back lost time. Yesterday is forever in the past and today is the only day we are guaranteed. We only have right now to change our lives. Why put of till tomorrow what you can do today?

So many of us are always saying, "Oh, well I'll start tomorrow," or, "I'll start Monday." Procrastination is something we all do and it is a hard habit to break. When your train of thought is to put things off because you always think you have time to do it later, you are just wasting those precious moments. There will never be a better time than now to change your life. If you need to, write out a pros and cons list of your current lifestyle compared to the version of yourself you want to be. You will see it is the absolute best decision you can make for yourself and those around you. I know your loved ones want you around for as long as possible, so do it for them too.

We have talked about all the reasons why people set a goal and never follow through with it. The people who have made the decision to change their life but quit far outnumber those who actually transform themselves. This is because they were not equipped mentally as you are now. They never understood their WHY or gained the knowledge. You now have all the tools to drastically change your life.

Will you accomplish your goals or let life pass you by? If you want to succeed, you need to set goals. Without goals you lack focus and direction. Goal setting will allow you to take control of your life's direction, the course you want to chart, to a healthier, fitter life. It also provides you with a benchmark for determining whether you are succeeding and meeting your goals. To accomplish your goals, you do need to know how to set goals. It's not realistic to say, "I want…" and expect it to happen. Goal Setting is a process that has to start with the WHY, and follow with details of what you want to accomplish. Yes, it will be hard work to actually accomplish it, but you are prepared this time, and you can apply what we shared with you in this book to accomplish your goals.

Here are some steps we have used for setting goals and accomplishing them.

1. Motivational Goals – Motivation is the key to accomplishing goals, so set a goal that will inspire you and motivate you. It

has to start with you and be the most important goal to start with. Reaching your goal should have a tremendous value for you. This once again is your WHY, so write it down. Why it is valuable and important to you to accomplish this goal?

2. Set Specific Goals – Your goal must be very clear, crystal clear, and very well defined. Write down where you want to end up, precisely to the point. If you are vague, you have a tendency to roam, so be specific and detailed.

3. Write down your goals on paper. Did you know the physical act of writing down a goal on paper makes it REAL and very tangible? It helps you visually SEE your goal and makes it much more realistic. It takes away the excuse of forgetting it because it's written down. Frame your goals in a positive manner. We add photos and motivational quotes to our goals when we write them. We also use a Goal Card, an affirmation card with an expiration date to hold ourselves accountable. Post your goals everywhere you can to visibly see them, to remind you of where you want to go. It will help you achieve your goals.

4. Take Action – Create a plan of action. Sometimes you become so focused on the goal that you miss this step and forget to plan. Plan your work and work your plan. I like to create a master plan of action, so I can track progress, cross off my to-do list. By making a plan and carrying it out with action you continuoulsy move closer to your goals.

5. Stay the course – Stick with it NO MATTER WHAT. You got this! Setting goals is truly an ongoing process. The struggles of life will come up and your willpower and determination will push you to persevere when times get tough.

Make the commitment today!

One tool we use to ensure we are taking action each day toward our goals is an affirmation page. It details what you will do on a daily basis to propel you toward your goals.

You will write down your own action steps you know you need

to take to accomplish your goals. You have to customize this to what works best for you. Every morning I wake up, go into my guest bedroom and look at my vision board with a dry erase board next to it. The dream board reminds me of my goals and my WHY, but the dry erase board is where I write my action steps. I most often write a new singular thought for each new day that I want to focus on. Or, if I'm struggling with one thing, I will make sure it's written on the board until I defeat it.

Put your affirmation page somewhere you have to look at it every morning you wake up. Put it on your desk at work, in your car, in your gym locker, on your refrigerator, EVERYWHERE! The more you are reminded of the thought process that aligns with your goals, the easier it is to fight of temptation and stay on track without derailing. Your affirmation page contains the action steps you will take every day. It keeps your why in front of your face so you never lose the reason you started this journey. The more you look at your affirmation page and do the things you set out to do, the more you give yourself a sense of strength. You challenge yourself to new heights you previously thought were not attainable.

What's stopping you?

Up until this point in your life, you have made excuse after excuse about why you are the way you are and how you will never be anything better. Today is the day to drop the stinkin thinkin and excuses to set forth on a course to accomplish your goals. Everyone is busy, everyone has a million irons in the fire, and yet some still find a way to go after their dreams. Remember, if it's important enough to you, you will find a way. Negativity does nothing but weigh you down and keep you from being the best version of yourself. You have to make a conscious decision TODAY to lose the negativity and become a more positive optimistic person. You can accomplish all you want in your health transformation, but you must first believe that you can. You can achieve whatever you set your mind to.

Starting today you have to eliminate the obstacles and make your goals a priority. You have to put yourself first. We have talked about how many people feel guilty and selfish when they spend time focusing on themselves. When you take time away from your family, children or even work to focus on your own priorities and goals, it can play mental games with you. The negative feelings associated with this mindset are what hold many back. Life balance has to be a focal point in your new transformation. You are living in this world too. You are not in this world just to serve everyone around you.

The happiness you gain from chasing your individual dreams is contagious, and what better message to spread to your friends and family than to chase your dreams. What an incredible life lesson to teach your children. The benefits do not stop there. The new you is more confident, has more energy and just has a higher sense of self-worth that carries over to all the other aspects of your life.

Why not you? Why do you not deserve to do this for yourself? Why are you not capable of being the healthiest fittest version of yourself you can possibly be? The answer to all those questions is, in fact, you deserve this and you absolutely can and will. We are proof that if you want to change your life, it is possible. We do not possess super-human willpower and incredible genetics that turn Oreos to muscle. We were just two overweight people from completely different walks of life who individually decided enough was enough. We made the decision to stop feeling sorry for ourselves and do something about it. Just as we have, you can too. The only thing stopping you is you. Your negative thought processes are holding you back.

Exercise 6:

Now write down what lifestyle changes you are going to put into practice to progress toward your goals. What is something negative in your life you need to rid yourself of to stay the course? What has stopped you in the past from accomplishing what you have always dreamed of?

Chapter 7

Lifelong Journey

Robby

My Toothpaste Analogy

When I first left college and moved back home, I bounced around a lot between churches. With my new mentality of personal growth, I wanted an environment that would challenge me. I finally settled on a great church with awesome people who both challenged me and allowed me to grow.

One question still remained from all the different churches I have visited—Which version of the Bible is the best one? I would ask a ton of people and get a different answer from everyone. I wasn't confused because I knew as long as I was spending time in some version of the Bible, I was taking action to better myself. But as we have talked about before, you want to put yourself in the optimal environment for growth.

I asked my preacher to coffee one morning because with my self-education, I developed questions he may be able to help me answer. So I asked him, "What version of the Bible do you recommend?" His immediate response was, "I can't." He could see the puzzled look on my face, so he elaborated and explained why he thought this way.

He told me something I would never forget, "If you went to the dentist and asked him which brand of toothpaste is the best, his response will be, 'Whichever one you will use the most.' You have to read and study the one you are going to use the most." After thinking about that profound statement, it made complete sense and I applied it to the rest of my life as well.

I am asked all the time which diet I recommend or what is the best way to burn calories, and I simply reply with this analogy. It does absolutely no good to go on a "diet" that you cannot stick to for the rest of your life. I don't even like using the word diet. I eat according to my goals. You have to discover through learning your body which foods and exercise work for you because you have to make a lifestyle change not just lose a little weight. The way you eat and work out have to be an evolving permanent change.

Most people set a goal weight "I just want to lose 20lbs." They start doing the latest fad diet and that is the extent of their healthy journey. They reach the point where they lose the weight and then they stop. While yes, losing the weight is a great accomplishment, we are talking about making this a permanent lifelong journey to health and fitness. Fad diets come and go with each new day and they only offer a temporary fix to what you're trying to accomplish. If you get stabbed, you don't put a Band-Aid on it and think that's going to help. You must make a permanent fix that will last you a lifetime. As in the previous chapter, we advocate learning not only nutrition and training methods but also learning how your body reacts to each. In order to make a lifelong change and to make this your new lifestyle, you must understand why you are doing what you're doing.

In the bigger picture of your health, yo-yo dieting actually does more harm than good. Drastically losing weight at a fast pace, then in most cases putting on more that you just lost, is a problem many suffer. In most cases it is because people start this new diet out there and then a month into it they realize they just cannot live like this anymore. After going six weeks of eating zero carbohydrates and only chicken, you realize there is no way you can maintain this for the rest of your life.

Karol

I firmly believe limits don't exist if you don't give them a reason.

While it is important to set goals and have short-term accomplishments, it is far more important to make this your new lifestyle. A healthy lifestyle does not have a destination. It is forever. It took both Robby and me many years to figure this out, for it to actually sink in, that it has to be a life change.

For years, it was a Band-Aid that we applied to cover up the wound but never actually addressed the real issues. It took me a few times of yo-yo dieting to realize that I needed to change my lifestyle for good, not for six weeks or six months, but for LIFE. I would lose some weight and feel great, but without changing my lifestyle and my eating habits, I would put it back on and gain more. It was a tough couple of years and I think how unhealthy it was for me.

Then, I made that change in 2008 and never looked back at the old me. I finally got it. I just understood and made the commitment that I wanted to live a healthy life. I never wanted to walk into another doctor's office and know that I am at the point where I now had serious health issues that I brought on myself from my unhealthy lifestyle. I never wanted to go more than two days without some form of exercise to help me get fit and healthy.

I also got help to understand why I was emotionally eating and addressed my feelings associated with that and what triggered it. It was time. It had all come full circle and in that moment, I knew the only way to stay on this healthy lifestyle was to truly commit to it, to leave the old me and my old habits in the past. From that day forward, I knew I needed to commit to a healthy and fit lifestyle.

Fast forward six years and I have stayed the course. Yes, it has been hard at times, but this new lifestyle is so rewarding to me. I FEEL great. My self-image is repaired, my self-esteem is sky rocketing, and I am stronger and leaner than I ever imagined I'd be.

I live in a city where we love to eat and we celebrate everything with food. Let's face it, it's the best food in the country (or at least I think so). It is a challenge to make healthy choices in my city of fabulous food. It is a challenge to wake up at 5:30 a.m. five times a week, and drive forty minutes to and from the gym. It is a challenge to go to the grocery store and pass up the bakery, but I got this. I am equipped with my Superman Cape, and my motivation and passion take me through it.

Do I splurge? Do I celebrate with food? Yes, of course I do. But, I balance it out with one cheat meal, not a day, week or season. I might work out thirty minutes more to burn up those calories, but I balance it out. The biggest thing is I don't eat with my emotions anymore. I enjoy food JUST as much as the next person, but I know the benefits of making healthy choices and there is no better feeling for me than this feeling of self-confidence, self-esteem and positive attitude be-cause I make healthy choices to get me closer to my goals.

Do not think about this new healthy lifestyle as a new diet or work out plan, you must think about it as a road map to accomplish your goals. You do not diet to lose weight; you simply eat according to what outcome you want. When you think nearsightedly such as a diet, it often becomes harder to follow through because you can allow nega-tivity to come into your life. When you are not focused on the bigger picture of your health, you lose the real reason why you should be doing this. Remember, vanity only has a short fuse of motivation. You have to retrain your brain to think about this as a process and a journey, versus a diet to get a few pounds off. A diet is nothing more than a short-term Band-Aid on a much larger problem—a way to lose quick weight but not the way to become the healthiest, strongest, version of you.

Healthy Lifestyle – A long-term commitment of eating right, exercising and becoming more emotionally fit. A healthy lifestyle is the new version of yourself that you always wanted to be.

We are all going to have moments of weakness or times when we think the task at hand may just be too hard. You may have a deadline at work that forces you to work late and miss your exercise for the day. Stumbling blocks are going to happen. They are just a part of being human. You may fall down, but the important part is to get back up and learn from it. When I think of perseverance, one story in particular comes to mind.

Arguably the greatest basketball player of all time did not even make his team the first time he tried out. Michael Jordan loved the game of basketball and ever since he was a little kid it was all he would do. But when he first tried out for his high school team, he did not even make the roster. After he read the posted roster and did not see his name on it, the disappointment set in. He went home to sulk, but when his mother saw him, she gave him just the words he needed to hear. "She said that the best thing I could do is to prove to the coach that he had made a mistake," recalled Michael. From this setback Jordan developed an unbelievable work ethic and determination to succeed. Michael owes his success to his level of commitment. While he did not like it, he learned to appreciate failure. At times when he is tired and just wants to quit, he reminds himself of his WHY through the vivid picture in his head of his name not being on the roster.

"I know that fear is an obstacle for some people, but for me it is just an illusion... Failure always makes me try harder on the next opportunity"
~ Michael Jordan

Just as Jordan learned the lesson of a lifetime through failure, you have to learn from your stumbles. The first place to start would be to understand why it happened in the first place. What is the underlying reason why you made that negative decision?

Part of this new, healthy lifestyle is understanding your desires and emotions. You have to understand why you make the decisions you make, and it is completely individual to every person. The importance of why you need to learn from your bad choices is so in the future you do not make the same mistakes again. Personal growth is a large part of this new healthy lifestyle and it will benefit every aspect of your life, but you must make the decision to not let mistakes affect you negatively. You must turn them around into something positive you can learn from. You also need to allow the positive things in your life to become anchors during the hard times.

Setbacks and challenges are inevitable. We are all human and yes, we all make poor choices from time to time. The most important thing is not to let that one bad decision of eating poorly on that holiday turn into a holi-week or holi-month. Do not give yourself a hall pass to extend the bad choice any longer. People start to think, "Oh I've been good. I can have that dessert or that cheat meal." While I'm not saying a cheat meal is bad, the problem comes when people extend a cheat meal into totally going off their new lifestyle because of it satisfying their need for immediate gratification. You have to isolate the bad choice, make sure it is only one bad choice, and get back on track immediately. It is so easy to let one bad decision compound to multiple bad decisions without even thinking about it.

Setbacks will happen. Even the strongest of us break weak every now and then. And, in a region where we celebrate everything with food, setbacks seem to come at us like bowling balls—fast and furious. From graduations, to Mardi Gras King Cake, to music festivals with some of the best food to enjoy, it is sometimes inevitable. I created some pretty sturdy "guardrails" to help me stay the course.

Even with my job, we always were celebrating a baby shower, birthday, promotion or entertaining clients. A lot of times were literally out of my control. And, food pushers, "Come on, have a piece of cake. Really, I am so offended you won't eat what I brought for potluck," or, "How can you live in this city and not eat that food."

Sometimes I would cave and I would mentally hit my guardrails to try and keep me on the healthy road.

One guardrail was to commit to exercise it off, literally thirty extra minutes on cardio to try and burn it off, and I was very true to that. I had to balance it. I had to take ownership of my setback and put my plan into action to compensate for it. My other guardrail was not to allow myself to turn this into "mental permission" to be wild and food free for many meals. It was a setback, an indulgence, for one meal, not for one whole day or the weekend, and I held myself accountable for it. I also tried to make a balanced healthy choice if I knew it was going to set me back. Meaning, if it was potluck, I would do a big salad so I could have the slice of King Cake and not eat the entire meal unhealthy. I would chart down what I ate, so I could see my setback, accept the responsibility and get ready to work it off the next day. My mental guardrails helped me stay on a very healthy, fit road.

That is why you have to stay conscious of the decision-making process and keep your why at the forefront of your mind. Use that as your motivation when making your next decision. It takes a lot of time, effort and hard work to progress toward your goals. You cannot let a series of bad decisions take away all the progress you just made. Next time you are in a situation where you know there is a high likelihood you are going to make a bad decision, most importantly think of your why but also think of all the hard work you put in to get to this point.

Setbacks can kill our morale. We can lose focus on how important this goal is to us. So that is why it is important to have others in your life who support your goals. It may not come from a spouse or a best friend but someone who understands the struggles and is on a similar journey. Sharing stories with like-minded individuals where you discuss your struggles and your successes will encourage not only you but them. It has a synergistic effect. It is often hard to do things alone in this world. A thorough support system to keep you accountable, motivated, and pick you back up when you fall is necessary. Remember to lean on your support system to get up and stay up.

I Found My Support System

That is why I joined Weight Watchers. I knew I needed a self-help group to share my struggle with, people who really were going through the same challenges I was when it came to over eating and not so much exercise. We all had different reasons why we struggled with food—emotional eating and stress eating like me, not wanting to cook and eating out a lot, or just not knowing a lot about nutrition. Everyone was there for a reason but we were there.

It was the BEST support system I could have ever asked for. Our Fearless Team Leader, Pam Davis, made it feel as if this meeting was just for you. She made it relatable to your challenges. I would look around and could see in everyone's face that they felt the same way. We would all nod our heads and agree. We would discuss our issues and hear stories from other members that would help get me through.

It was my backbone to building a better me and every Sunday morning at 9 a.m. WW school was in session, and there I was in the front row with Sylvia, learning about nutrition and what foods really are good for you. Learning about portion control (yeah, that was a hard one) and looking at six ounces, saying, "Wow, I have been consuming three times as much!" We were all educating ourselves with the knowledge we needed to make better choices and addressing the hard stuff—the emotional part of eating for me.

Just like AA, we all let it out, from tears of sadness to tears and celebration of joy when someone would reach a milestone. That could be losing five pounds to losing fifty pounds to losing one hundred pounds. We were all there to support one another, week in and week out and if the scale tipped the other way, we too, were there to encourage and support one another.

I had twenty plus supporters in one room. How lucky I was to be surrounded by like-minded people who were all there to retrain their brains so they too could change the course of their life to a healthy, fit, lifestyle. I do keep in touch with some of the members. Some of them go to the same gym as me.

In Alcoholics Anonymous, you go through all the steps to recognize you have a problem and how to fix the problem. It is a great starter to kick off your sobriety, but the most important lesson to learn from AA and the most important thing they do to keep people sober is form support groups and assign everyone a sponsor. When you are assigned a sponsor, you call this person when you get the urge where you just have to have that drink and you are feeling week. It is the sponsor's responsibility to bring you back from the ledge. The sponsor coaches you on why it is important to not make that bad decision and then helps you realize why you have the desire to make that bad decision.

When someone makes a decision, constant feedback is a very good way to keep the train on the tracks. Surrounding yourself with other people on the same journey as you who can provide feedback will actually help you follow through with your goals. Having a source of constant feedback is crucial to your journey. Feedback comes in many forms from a co-worker asking if you lost weight to your best friends asking why you are so happy today. Just something as simple as those two questions provide us with a sense of accomplishment. They tell us what we are doing is working and others can see it. We are often our own worse critics and we can judge ourselves very harshly. Getting feedback from someone you know and trust can help you rid yourself of your negative thinking. Just like AA, find a sponsor or a friend, anyone who can be there for you and provide you with that much-needed feedback.

You can learn from the addiction recovery model and implement it into your new, healthy lifestyle. Numerous studies have proved that food leads to a chemical reaction, just like alcohol and drugs, and it feeds the same desires and emotions as addiction does. We both can look back now and say food was our choice of drug, our addiction. We were dealing with emotions and some voids in our lives. Instead of turning to drugs, we turned to food. Food became what we turned to any time negative emotions entered our thought processes. Just like an alcoholic needed a drink, we needed a pizza, a whole pizza.

Just like any addiction, you are taking a negative thought process and compounding it with a negative decision, which starts a negative spiral. Unless you understand the signs and symptoms of what starts the spiral, you can get trapped in it. Before you know it, it has completely affected every aspect of your life. This is why personal growth is so important. You have to understand your triggers and learn not to give in to them in future.

The next time you feel the need to make a decision that is counterproductive to your goals, take a step back and evaluate the situation. Remember, we are focusing on long-term benefits versus giving in to impulses and urges. It takes on average about three minutes for a food craving to pass. Instead of giving in to the craving, do something productive that will take your mind off of it such as going for a short walk or doing some stretching in your office. After you take your mind off of it, it is helpful to come back and think through the situation. Am I stressed? Am I dehydrated? When was the last time I ate healthy foods? What caused the craving in the first place? Once you isolate the cause, you can start to reprogram yourself not to fall victim to those impulse decisions again.

In order to make this the start of your journey, here are the action steps you need to take to ensure success in reaching your goals. Take time to write down your personal E.V.O.L.V.E. challenge.

"Your brain is the first muscle you must get in shape."

1. *E* valuation – You have to evaluate your mindset and emotions to prepare yourself for the journey ahead. Get rid of your negative self-image and your insecurities. You have unlimited potential to accomplish all you set out to accomplish if you tear down that wall of negativity. What in your life is holding you back? What are some negatives in your life you need to rid yourself of?

2. *V* ision and WHY – Once you rid yourself of the negatives, it is time to focus on what you want. What does this journey look like to you? What outcomes do you wish to achieve? Now visualize yourself doing it and visualize what positives will come out of this new you. Write down your vision and clearly define what you want to accomplish and why.

Discover your WHY. Why do you want to make this change in your life? What is your internal motivation? The why will supply you with the motivation not only to get you started, but also your Why will get you through your struggles along your journey.

3. *O* nward – Do not overcomplicate and bog down this decision. The key is that you start moving toward your goals. What are you going to implement in your life to ensure success? How are you going to make a change today to start your new life? What commitment are you going to make to yourself today to change your life?

4. *L* earn Your Body – You have to educate yourself. During your new healthy lifestyle journey, you are going to grow on the inside just as much as you do on the outside. You are going to learn how to eat, what to eat and even how your body responds to certain types of food as part of the educational process. Becoming the healthiest version of you involves learning how to optimize your body. You will learn many lessons along the way, and the educational process is perpetual. Keep a transformation log with notes on energy levels, what you ate, what you did for exercise, and any negatives you are dealing with.

5. *V* alor – is defined as boldness, determination and courage. You now know why you are wanting to do this, and you have how you are going to do this through self-education. Now it is the time to move confidentially in the direction of your dreams. You are armed with everything you need, and there is nothing left to do, but to do it. Persist until you succeed! How will you stay strong in this new lifestyle? What will you do to overcome obstacles?

6. *E* njoy Yourself – Find joy in this new lifestyle. Find meals and exercise plans you actually enjoy doing. The more you enjoy the process the more likely you are to stick to it. While we believe there is joy in the process, the ultimate joy comes from achieving your goals. What are you going to do to ensure you make this a lifelong journey?

The Struggle is Real

Complete the E.V.O.L.V.E. challenge.

Chapter 8

Enjoy Your New Lifestyle

Robby

Passion – a strong or extravagant fondness, enthusiasm,
or desire for something better

The passion you develop from the journey of becoming a new healthier you is built on the struggles you have overcome. As you progress on your journey, you are going to go through many battles as we have discussed. The Struggle Is Real because we are human beings living in the real world. We are not some robot that has zero emotions and feelings. We develop strong emotions throughout our lives. Often those emotions are spurred by tough times. Becoming the healthiest you mentally and physically will be tough. At times you will want to give up and go back to your old ways, but persevering through these tough times will develop your passion for this new lifestyle. After you have achieved a short-term goal, you get excited and think about all the hard work it took. It makes you stronger and ready to tackle the next challenge.

Your passion can transcend yourself and inspire others. It will be an outpouring of emotions and enthusiasm that we promise will be very noticeable to those around you. People will see a little extra bounce in your step and a new brighter smile on your face because you have now come to the realization that if you can do it, so can those around you. Passion and energy are contagious. You are now being a healthier positive version of yourself and you will want everyone to join in with you on the journey. The saying "The more the merrier" is very true in the world of health and fitness.

The passion is very noticeable with Karol and me. You can hear it in the way we talk and even the way we carry ourselves. It is plastered all over on our social media. Our mutual passion for fitness is how we first met.

Karol

The Power of Two – we joined forces to inspire.

I am convinced people come into your life for a reason, and I am convinced that I met Robby's friend Chase so Robby and I could write this book. As you read this book and progress on your own transformation, there will be people who will journey with you every step of the way, and then there will people who will be by your side for what I call a short trip—like a road trip. Robby is the former. As soon as I met him, I knew we would be on a lifelong journey together for a reason.

I met Robby the first time through a mutual friend at a concert in Baton Rouge. We were there to see one of our favorite bands, Otherwise (who knew we both liked rock and roll). I was with my then boyfriend, now husband, Colin and Robby was with Chase. It was a huge night of rock for us, and I was decked out to the T. I was feeling amazing and my self-esteem was so back. I treated myself that day with hair and makeup by the most awesome stylist, Gabby. I felt like a queen and I just carried myself so confidently that night because my clothes fit well (no tugging), I felt beautiful and I was with my sweetie going to see one of our favorite bands.

Chase and his friends were meeting us there and as always he showed up a little late. We were already standing in the front, but they came and found us. Chase introduced us to Robby and another friend Jeff, both very nice guys and both with very nice builds. You could tell they worked hard for it, ate right and exercised, and it gave me an instant feeling of respect as I stood near them feeling the same way. I was confident because I have worked hard on me from the inside out, from the self-image on the inside to my appearance on the outside, and my self-esteem showed.

Robby stood near us a the concert, and we had a few girls who'd had a few too many and ironically started giving me and my friend, Jeanne the evil eye. We still think to this day they must have liked Robby and his friends and they thought we were with them. So, in the middle of the stare down, I went over to Robby and said, "Security, I think I need you to break this up." He took pride in me calling him and Jeff security, so they came over and hung out by us the rest of the night. We didn't talk a whole lot that night because we were at a rock show—a loud one and awesome one at that. Afterward, we had a chance for all of us to talk a bit more. I left that night thinking how great it was to meet some new friends who loved rock as much as we did.

The next time I saw Robby was at another concert in Biloxi, and he came very early this time. I was working for his friend at the time, so I too was early to the event. We seized a chance to talk, the normal stuff, how are you, how is Colin, how's work, where are you from, etc. I had a hot pink sleeveless shirt on that night and I have to say, my arms and shoulders were looking super lean and muscular, and I was feeling just as confident about myself that night as when I met Robby. He made a comment about a how hard I must work out to stay in such good shape and I thought, "You must work out too." He had on a tight fitted shirt and you could see he exercised. He was very physically fit.

So, we immediately started talking, and yes, my name should be chatty Karol because I do love to talk, especially about health and fitness. We talked about what type of exercises we do, where we work out, our meal plans, etc. and we shared what we both do to stay motivated. I then told Robby some of my story—that I wasn't always this way. I lost over one hundred pounds six years ago and now enjoy a very happy, healthy and fit lifestyle. He stopped, literally a long pause between two people who love to talk, looked down at the ground, and almost embarrassed, lifted his head and said, "Karol, I too have lost over one hundred pounds and have kept it off and now lead a very healthy, fit lifestyle."

Needless to say I don't remember much of the concert because for a few hours (it felt like it), we shared our Struggles with one another and finally, I had someone to talk with who **REALLY** walked in my shoes, got what I went through, went through it himself and came out a new person, ready to inspire and motivate people. I told him how my boyfriend had written a book, Dream Training, and how Colin had encouraged me to write a book (and yes, watching him write and publish his third edition was so beyond inspiring to me) about my transformational weight loss and healthy lifestyle journey. I told him I had been wanting to write it to inspire others who were going through the Struggle. We immediately started bouncing ideas back and forth. We talked about how you must first change your mindset, then change your body and eating habits. I did it the natural way and old-fashioned way, retraining my brain and my body.

Robby once again stopped me, but this time, with a **HUGE** smile on his face and said, "Karol, me too. I have been wanting to write my transformational weight loss journey and share it with the world to motivate people and let them know that with the resources out there today, it is possible." So, I said, "Robby, we need to write this book together." And Robby said, "Yes, we will!" That night we started sharing ideas on how to collaborate and share our struggles. We also talked about how we overcame those struggles to live a healthy, fit lifestyle.

The passion we share is what drove us to write this book and want to pour into other people all we have learned and continue to learn each new day. Our passion to inspire others, like YOU, is contagious and so motivating and we hope you have truly felt our passion, page by page! While we know we are not experts in the fields of nutrition or exercise, and we definitely do not claim to be psychologists, we understand the struggles of this change. We have coupled our own knowledge and learned through endless interviews and countless hours of research on various topics with regards to this book.

How we continue to stay passionate is by inspiring others when we are able to pour into others and see the change in them. Trying to be the light to others started well before this book was even an idea. We just enjoyed this new lifestyle and what it produced in us so much that we wanted to tell everyone. We knew that while we were making an impact to those closest to us, we still yearned to reach as many people with this message as we could.

As you progress on your journey, you will be changing from the inside out. Your self-image will grow stronger with each new challenge and goal you reach. As you go shopping because none of your clothes fit, as your doctor tells you that you are no longer a risk for diabetes or even need blood pressure medicine, you will gain confidence in your ability to tackle problems and handle adversity. You realize you have just done the best thing for yourself you possibly could and it will empower you to welcome new challenges because you realize how strong of a person you really are.

"I firmly believe that any man's finest hour, the greatest fulfillment of all that he holds dear, is that moment when he has worked his heart out in a good cause and lies exhausted on the field of battle — victorious."
~ Vince Lombardi

The purpose of this book is to make you feel better about yourself. We say it over and over and here it is again, yes, this is about YOU. It is about building your self-image and self-esteem giving you confidence and motivation, which when all combined, is unstoppable. Hopefully it also catches on to ones around you who support the new, healthy, fit, and happy you! Once you have built that self-esteem, you truly begin to see so many benefits of this healthy lifestyle you deserve for yourself. Stop and celebrate your successes, celebrate reaching your goals with something positive. You can go buy some new clothes, go on a trip, pamper your body, go do a spa day with your gym buddies or do something for you to pay it forward. It's your moment and you have worked so very hard to get there. So, yes, bask in the sun, and really thank yourself! There really is no better feeling than fighting through the struggles to accomplish your goals.

I lived with a relentless pursuit of better, and I believe it's important to celebrate your success!

In order for me to fully enjoy this new lifestyle, I had to correct some internal issues first.

Over time and many years of yo-yo dieting, emotional eating, and being in unhealthy relationships, my self-image was beaten down. The image tattooed in my head was the version of myself at my heaviest. The image of me being so overweight that you could barely see my eyes when I took pictures because my face was so big. That image assured my self-esteem was the smallest part of me. I once had a boyfriend tell me that I looked like the Michelin mummy. He said that I was so big and round, I walked like him, oh, and the Pillsbury Doughboy too, which of course, I had to eat my share of cinnamon rolls that week to emotionally get over the hurt and the pain of those comments

It was how I had begun to see myself. It was the perception I formed by being told and believing I was not pretty at all. Many experts will tell you, you begin forming your perception of your attractiveness, health, acceptability and functionality in early childhood. If that was the case with me, I was a cheerleader, on Prom Court, Dance Team, gymnast, as a child I thought I was very healthy, actually really muscular and pretty.

With time and from the feedback of others, I started to self-criticize. I developed a very negative internal image of my body. I began to internalize this, and my perception of my own beauty created a negative body image because I regularly criticized myself and others joined in. I have to say, this was just as hard as losing the one hundred pounds. This weighed heavier on me than the weight did.

I share this story with you because I know that struggle, and it was truly one of the lowest moments in my life. My self-image was right there at the bottom, and I knew it had become a disorder and I had to dig deep and crawl out of it. I did…and so can you!

It took some time and some unpeeling of the emotions, but I addressed why I emotionally ate and why my self-image was so beaten down. I had to actually own it. I had to recognize and acknowledge my feelings and what I needed to do to stop suppressing them.

My dad gave me an article at the time that talked about grit. After reading it I know this is when I needed to dig deep and remind myself that yes, I could change my self-image. The article said

"Grit is defined as indomitable courage, toughness and resolution."
~ Linda Cuccia, Metro Fitness

Grit is what it takes to move when you do not feel like moving. I lived by this quote and it is now tattooed in my brain instead of my negative self-image. One day at a time, in the midst of the struggle and fixing myself, I addressed my feelings and emotions head on. I began to look at myself in the mirror again and love me again for me, no matter what size I was at the time. With the help of my friends and family, Weight Watchers group, eating right and exercising (and yes, me and the not-so-nice boyfriend split up), I started to focus on my perception of my body and fix my self-image. It took years—a very, very, very long and slow process—to really repair and rebuild my self-image.

I did it and now it was better than before. I finally began to love myself again, for ME. I began to tell myself positive affirmations over and over again and guess what, I started to believe them and SEE the real me again. I would say to myself, "I love and accept me for me, unconditionally." I feel great about myself and my new healthy, fit lifestyle. I have high self-esteem as I now respect myself. I deserve to look in the mirror and see all that hard work is paying off. I release any misery and suffering, change it into a positive, and think happy thoughts.

FINALLY, I was comfortable in my own skin.

After six-plus years of reinforcing my strong self-image, the moment came that led to me enjoying my new life full-circle. It was July 19th, 2015. At my wedding, the biggest rock wedding ever. I stood up on stage, in my custom corset wedding dress, saying I do to my most handsome King, my husband Colin. For the first time in six-plus years, I finally loved BEING IN MY OWN SKIN. I felt comfortable and confident in my own skin. Seeing and loving myself again, I could visibly see the positive radiance flowing out of me.

In that moment on stage, saying our vows, I did not waiver, I did not flinch, I did not tug at my corset. I did not say or look at myself in a negative way. Nope, not today, not ever again. In this moment, I was Superwoman Karol, I was 100% enjoying my new life, and my self -image was back. I never felt better about myself. For that day, July 19th…I did hold my head up high. I did smile uncontrollably. I did have a tight fitting dress that I felt very confident in wearing. I did work hard mentally, and yes, a lot of sweat, physically to get to this day. I did make healthy food choices and made better decisions to get to this day. I did look at myself in the mirror in my wedding dress. Then I wanted to see myself in pictures from my wedding day. Most of all, I did it, my self-image had been restored. Personally feeling this was the best feeling of my life.

I have seen so many benefits of my "new life' with my self-image restored. My self-esteem and confidence level is off the charts. I feel so much healthier, so much fitter, and I have so much more energy. My health is at its peak. My recipe for a healthy body: drink lots of water, take my vitamins, eat clean and exercise, get a good night of sleep, and then repeat! I have to do all of these actions every day in order to reach my goal. I feel great in my clothes, I actually FEEL great in my clothes. That was a MILESTONE for me, and you too will FEEL that way.

I also see this overflow into my professional world as I am more confident and I can actually see how this new life has directly contributed to my success. This year alone, I have built back my confidence to start my own business again and be that entrepreneur I long to be. I am positive and full of self-confidence when I walk into a meeting now. I love making eye contact, smiling and carrying myself in a very positive mindset. It's noticeable and people tell me. They ask, "What you are doing? You look great!" Which leads me to the part of my new lifestyle that I enjoy the most, sharing my story and motivating others. It is a huge benefit for me as I really enjoy passing on my lifestyle changes and how enjoyable it is living a healthy, fit, lifestyle.

I also have someone to share my healthy, fit, lifestyle who shares the same passion for living it every day. My husband Colin has helped me in more ways than he will ever know. His commitment to fitness and eating healthy is a part our everyday life. He exercises every day, makes great healthy choices, and encourages and supports me along the way. The journey is even more enjoyable when I can share my passion and my new lifestyle with someone who has the same commitment as me. We are always searching for new information, new health products, new exercises and good, tasty recipes for us to stay the course and enjoy doing this together.

Also, my parents are truly my biggest inspirations. My dad, at the age of eighty, is still very active and works out regularly. My mother, in her late seventies, just stopped playing competitive tennis but still walks and stays very active. And, they make very healthy choices with their food and nutrition. They are the prodigy of what living a healthy, active lifestyle looks like, and I enjoy sharing my new lifestyle with them. They are there to encourage and support me as well.

I now challenge you to Pay It Forward. We want you to spread this message to help others. Through this transformational journey, you will be required to make sacrifices and changes that will be hard at times. The struggles will force you to become a better person than you ever thought possible. Now is your time to pass along all of your newfound strength. After all it is better to give than too receive. Share your story with others.

We have a community of people like you on Facebook under #TheStruggleIsReal. Here you can share with others and find strength in others if you need it. It is your community to support you along your journey. You can ask for help with anything pertaining to your transformation and others who have had the same struggles will be there to respond and give you encouragement. Most importantly it is your platform to share your successful transformation story with the hash tag #ShareYourStory. It will not only feel good for you to tell the world what you have just accomplished but also think of all the others who will be inspired by your story. Your story may be the deciding factor that helps that one person change their life. The community can also be an easy way to find others around your location to form a support group. Not only will you have an online community as a resource but now you will have a #TheStruggleIsReal local group that you can meet with face to face.

One thing you can do that really makes your new lifestyle an absolute joy is to bring others with you along the way. Find someone you know could benefit from the lessons you have now learned and pour into them. Everyone could use an act of kindness. If you have a friend you know needs some help, you can buy them a copy and invite them with you on the journey. It is far easier to stick to this new lifestyle if you have someone right there with you through the struggles. During your transformation, you will, at times, be required to be selfish with your time and resources, but this is the reason why. You can now take this positive in your life and pay it forward. Spread the word and encourage others. As good as it feels to become healthy, it feels even better to help those nearest to your heart.

Robby

Your new lifestyle has to be enjoyable or it will not last. If you dread the process by constantly thinking how much you hate the food or how much you hate the exercise, then what is the likelihood of you continuing it for the rest of your life? While playing college football, I hated the constant conditioning and often dreaded practice because of my negative mindset. I dreaded the alarm clock going off because I knew it was going to be another day of endless running, lifting weights and getting my body battered and bruised. I thoroughly enjoyed each and every game, just not all the preparation for it. Now I have a completely different mindset. I work out because I want too. I genuinely enjoy the process and the way it makes me feel. I enjoy seeing the gradual changes of losing a little fat here or building a little muscle there.

I also enjoy finding new ways to make unhealthy recipes that I love healthy and enjoyable without the guilt. I will have a craving for something and my mind immediately goes to how I can I make this at home but be healthy. Why can't I have the foods I want but still be healthy? It is just another way I have found to enjoy this new lifestyle. My mother is often my guinea pig when I am experimenting with new recipes because she now enjoys the healthy lifestyle as well. Just this morning I made her stop by my house to try out a new muffin recipe I have been working on. She loved them and immediately asked me for the recipe. One of my favorite foods I have always loved is cheesecake. After a few batches and some trial and error, now I can make a high protein, low sugar and low fat cheesecake that tastes just like the real thing. I enjoy the fact I can show others that being healthy is not about sacrifice. It's about gain. You gain so much more value to your life than that piece of sugary fattening cheesecake. Think about it. How much better would life be if you were healthier mentally and physically?

You have to look at each new day with vigor to go and tackle the day with enjoyment. This life is meant to be lived, not simply to exist in it. With all the work you have been doing to better yourself, you can now apply that newfound confidence to your everyday life. Your transformation will have a spillover effect on all the other aspects of your life as well. Your new lifestyle will be enjoyable because you are changing inside and out. You are becoming healthy, and the feeling associated with knowing that you are taking care of your body is amazing. If you have taken the time to root out any negativity and problems in your head and focused on having a healthier body, you will see your work, your family life, your relationships all change for the better. Now that you have made yourself happy, it's time to make those around you happy. Happiness is very contagious to those who are seeking it.

We have given you some examples of how we have joy and fulfillment in our new healthy lifestyles, but you have to find your own sense of joy. Think about what benefits you are now seeing in your life. What are some of the challenges you have overcome that fill you with pride? How has your surrounding life improved since you have improved yourself? Your personal sense of joy will have meaning to you and you alone. What it will do is give you another motivating factor to continue the journey and progress even further. We have helped you get through the mental clutter and make a change in your life, but it is up to you to find the enjoyment that will make this a life long journey.

It may give you the confidence to go and pursue your real passions. After all, you have already conquered the hardest part—yourself. We have talked about the strength you gain from successful challenges. So where else in your life can you apply this new empowered you? What are your passions in life you have always been too insecure and fearful to chase? Apply the same lessons you have learned on your journey toward your passions. We would have never had the confidence to stand tall and write this book if we had not been through what we have. We have experienced the overwhelming peaks and the valleys we thought we would never get through. Through it all we were both working full-time jobs and had a lot going on, so the struggle was real at times. Those struggles gave us the passion and confidence to help others. We became stronger with each new challenge to the point where we now had the confidence to really chase our dreams. Our dreams just happened to be the same. One quote we kept in front of us throughout the writing of this book is:

"I want to inspire people. I want someone to look at me and say,
'Because of you I didn't give up.'"

Exercise 8:

You need to explore yourself to find your individual interests that you can see yourself enjoying along the journey. Is it cooking? Is it a workout class? Is it finding creative ways to be more active? Is it identifying the people and the support system that will help you along the way? Write down what you are going to implement in your life to enjoy this new journey.

Now, it's your turn. It's time for you to dream again. Take control of your life to make it look like what you want it to. Do not accept someone else's reality as your own. What do you want to accomplish? What is something you have always wanted but just never went for it? Start by changing yourself and then change the world around you. Pay it forward.

Through our journey we hope to inspire others. We want you to learn from our struggles and recognize them in your own life so you can E.V.O.L.V.E into the person you dream to be.

We are on this journey together, side by side, standing strong!

#TheStruggleIsReal

Thank you so much from the bottom of our hearts for reading our book. We want to help you reach and achieve your goals in any way we possibly can. We hope when you put down The Struggle Is Real, you will pick up the 30-Day E.V.O.L.V.E. Challenge Journal to cement this lifestyle change into a permanent journey into the new, healthy, motivated positive you. We are going to spell out the game plan in the book, but the journal walks you through how to implement it into your life. Also sign up for coaching sessions with the authors to allow them to pour into you and guide you through the mental transformation, so you can transform your body.

Acknowledgements

A Special Thanks To From Karol Brandt-Gilmartin

To my parents, Marilyn and Lloyd Brandt, for your unconditional love and support

To my sisters, Karen, Kim, Kathryn and Cathy for always there to lift me up, and always by my side

To My King, my husband Colin Gilmartin, for being my fearless mentor and who really encouraged me to write this book, share my story and follow in his Author Footsteps, I love you, thank you for your guidance and unwaivering love and helping me make my dream come to life

To my most beautiful, kind spirited daughter, Amanda Michelle Sullivan Owen for being such a ray of light in my life, always, I love you and for her father, Gary in teaching me how to be fearless

To my Gymnastics Coach Tara Schwegmann and my Weight Watchers Leader, Pam Davis for believing in me and always reminding me that yes, anything is possible

For Dr. Rose who made me "Fix Me"

For all of my friends and family, wayyyyy too many to name, who have seen me at every size and weight, big and small, who never left my side, always encouraging me and who always believed in me, supported me

To all the Rockers out there, thank you for producing kick ass rock n roll that I could get lost in all the time to sooth my soul, and focus on me to push me to reach my goals

And God, who will never forsake me, who is everlasting, his calling for me to write this book with Robby. I am so blessed to be able to share my story, I want to Pay It Forward for his will

A Special Thanks from Robby D'Angelo

I want first and foremost thank God for instilling in me the strength to go through the struggles and for all of the unanswered prayers because he knew his plan for me.

Mom and Dad, I would not be the man I am today without your enduring love and incredible example you set for me. Thank you so much for all of your support along my journey it meant more to me than you will ever know.

To my brothers who I know beyond a shadow of doubt have and always will be there no matter what.

The rest of my family; from my grandparents aunts and uncles to the many cousins who have helped raise me with all the love and support I could ever ask for.

To my friends "The Foxes" who have been like brothers to me since our days of playing college football together. Thank you all for your constant banter and reality checks. #July10

To Chase, Hughie and Jeff for propelling me to the next level in life and always providing motivation and support to ensure we all grow together. #MakeMovesOrMakeExcuses

I want to especially thank all of my teachers coaches and mentors that have influenced every facet of my life. Coach Ross, Coach Black,

Coach Bentz, Coach Sikes, Coach Rod, and Coach Bower thank you for pushing me on the field and truly showing me the capabilities everyone has inside of them if they are just willing to push a little harder. Mike Landrum thank you for opening my eyes to incredible teachings and business philosophies that I still carry with me and implement in my life.

To all the people along my journey who I have bugged and pestered about health and fitness. All of the gym rats who without even knowing push me to work harder because I see your grind. The fitness community for providing never ending support and motivation and especially the Fitness YouTubers: Christian Guzman, Steve Cook, Jerry Ward, Nick Wright, Elliot Hulse, Marc Lobliner, Chris Jones and Nick Wright just to name a few of the many I subscribe to and follow.

Lastly, I want to thank my struggle! Yes, I am thankful for all the negatives and crap I have been through because without them I would have the strength and determination. Without my struggles not have the opportunity in front of me to inspire others to achieve their dreams.

A Special Thanks from BOTH Robby and Karol

Jesse Krieger, our amazing Publisher for inspiring us to write it and let him handle the rest and he so did, thank you Jesse for all of your effort into making this book come to life!

Made in the USA
Middletown, DE
21 December 2015